12 DATES WITH AUTISM AND THE HOLY SPIRIT

NANA KODWO ADENTWI

FOREWORD BY REV. J. F. K. MENSAH

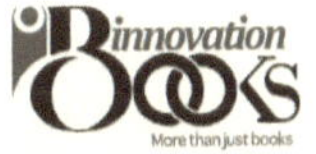

DEDICATION

I dedicate this book to my sons, Yooku Sompa, Siisi Siarfo and Fiifi Nkunyim.

May the HOLY SPIRIT continue to use them to hold our heads (my wife and I) above the rough waters of living with autism.

ACKNOWLEDGMENTS

I am forever grateful to the Holy Spirit for His guiding presence in my life.

My many precious thanks for this work go to my Sheila, my ever young wife for all the encouragement and beautiful additions.

I am very grateful to Mrs Muriel Acquaah Harrison, Dr Mrs Abena Tetteh, and Dr Nana Akua Owusu for all their inputs and encouragement to have this work finished and published.

I also thank Mrs Salomey Bekoe for all the secretarial work done to produce this book, and Mr Daniel Adapoe for the cover design and art symbols used in this book.

I am most particularly grateful to Reverend JFK Mensah for writing the instructive Foreword.

And to all the team at Print Innovation for all their creative additions and printing of this book.

CONTENTS

"A wonderful book with tools shared from the experiences of a Christian parent with positive outcomes over autism. It discusses the power and work of the Holy Spirit in daily living. A recommended good read with practical guidance to help our understanding and response to the global puzzle of autism. Read this book for inspiration and an emphasis on trusting in God's sovereign will."

By **Rev. Frank Gaisie,** Senior Pastor, Destiny Chapel, & Convenor, Hour of Destiny Prayer Network, UK.

"Definitely a book about autism, but much more than that. This is about a father's walk of faith with the Lord and love for his son. In this book, readers will encounter profound statements by the author, such as 'the innocence of children living with autism and their responses to little acts of kindness is in itself an emphatic revelation that they deserve acceptance, love and support'. Nana Kodwo recounts challenges of his family's association with autism, and like the hallowed Apostle Paul, enables us see how through our humanity we can appreciate the strengthening power of the Holy Spirit. He shows so much conviction in the empowerment of patience and understanding for all God's children, be they smart or slow, able or not so able. If you desire to be an expression of God's love to humans who find themselves with developmentally challenging circumstances, kindly read this book."

By **Loretta Roberts (Mrs)**, Civil & Environmental Engineer, UNICEF, Ghana.

FOREWORD

*Now as Jesus passed by, He saw a man who
was blind from birth. And His disciples asked Him,
saying, "Rabbi, who sinned, this man or his parents,
that he was born blind?" Jesus answered, "Neither
this man nor his parents sinned, but that the works of
God should be revealed in him. (**John 9:1-3 NKJV**)*

Every autobiography is rich because it is loaded with unforgettable experiences, real life encounters and memoirs that weigh more than any fiction. Biographies, autobiographies and memoirs of Christians are even richer because they often share the journey of the suffering righteous in fellowship with the Holy Spirit. *12 Dates With Autism And The Holy Spirit* is one such book. It overflows with encouragement for distressed parents of autistic children, illustrations of God's presence and explanations for our most difficult moments. The author is a practicing Christian for over four decades. He is married to Sheila and serves as an advocate for children with autism. You should listen to him share lessons imprinted upon their souls as a result of nurturing an autistic son for nearly twenty years. His recollections of the reality of the Holy Spirit as a Helper is so fresh.

The twenty-first century and much more our current generation has observed an upsurge in the cases of children diagnosed with autism spectrum disorder

(ASD). Families with autistic children suffer emotional distress, chaotic and confusing moments as the children manifest their autistic challenges. They engage in distractions and disrupt family activities. Some of these children frequently hurt themselves and engage in dangerous play. Living with this condition is the canvas-setting on which this book is painted. The ASD condition demands a myriad of special responses and interventions to constructively socialize and train the affected persons. But so much of these responses and approaches to raising autistic children in particular by their parents and guardians ought to be internally motivated and spiritually sustained. This book provides a searchlight and some leads towards practising and achieving success in that direction.

From a personal perspective as a believer, Nana Adentwi points to spiritual insights, promptings and wisdom from the Holy Spirit in dealing with both the emotional distress and confusing situations that the manifestations of autism presents to families and the affected children themselves. This is real. This is authentic. This is Christian. He describes and discusses the challenges that autism brings to the affected children and their families, and suggests interventions and internalized spiritual responses that could be deployed to manage and overcome them. The challenges dealt with include sleeplessness, heartaches, confusion and misguided thoughts, chaos, bewildering uncertainties, fears and trepidation. He stresses the point that managing autistic behavior and effecting correctional change involves a lot of role modelling, and hence the importance of teaching and nurturing positive attitudes in the affected children. The illustrations in this book show how relying on and drawing from the power of the Holy Spirit borne in His fruit, particularly faith, hope, peace and love can achieve positive attitudes and character formation in both the children and their parents.

There is an epilogue which provides a synopsis of selected Adinkra symbols, customarily original to the Akan people of Ghana, which speak to virtues, philosophies and beliefs that inspire resilience and an outlook to ultimate success in life. This is included to help affected families customize their deliberate responses to the challenges of autism, and to maintain their orientation to never give up on the fight to unearth the positive abilities buried in their children.

12 Dates With Autism And The Holy Spirit will do four things for you. It will school you in what children with autism and their parents go through. It will also give you empathy and admiration for parents with disabled children. Then it will arm you with effective tools to counsel ever-complaining Christian parents. Above all, it will help you appreciate and listen more closely to the Holy Spirit in life's worst moments.

Have you ever wondered whether God is the God of the disabled? Here is a book that provides rare answers from God's Spirit for parenting children with handicaps. Every chapter deals with an area of frustration that frequently hits the parent of an autistic child. Nana Kodwo skillfully weaves the Holy Spirit's comfort to him personally into an Adinkra tapestry of God's consolation to every questioning Christian caregiver. This book will challenge every parent to love your child despite everything.

If you faint in the day of adversity, your strength is small. **Prov.24:10**

By Rev. J.F.K. Mensah.

General Overseer, *Great Commission Church International*

President, *Christlike Disciplemakers Movement*

Rector, *Great Commission Bible School.*

INTRODUCTION

"Sometimes in this life, we suddenly come to a place where confusion and stress appear to be taking over, and yet we know we cannot give up because we love and treasure the life and joy of the subject of our pain. Then we come to another place when we climb a ladder from the dark night of the soul to the brilliance of God's glory. We may pass from a sense of abject alienation through confession and cleansing, to reconciliation and communion with God. These are the memorable experiences to which people refer back and draw consolation".

Culled from Morris Inch in his book, ***A Case For Christianity****, 1997.)*

This book is a memoir of living with autism. The chapters recount my first hand experiences, understanding and unique reflections on the manifestations of autism as I have observed them largely in the life of my dear son Yooku, and minimally from some of his peers in his special school in Accra, Ghana. Readers will find herein, very personal stories of the mystery, confusion, frustration, anxiety and anguish that living with autism brings to individuals and families. You will also find some expressions of my thoughts as well as beautiful moments (Kairos) of unction from the Holy

Spirit that have provided me and my family the strength and hope to keep on loving and supporting our son through his somewhat tough life.

As an individual and young parent, I knew almost nothing about autism when my son was diagnosed as a child on the autism spectrum. I had heard of the condition before. I had actually seen two children, sons of two friends of mine known to be on the autism spectrum. But the diagnosis of my son left me bewildered and in total denial. For the sake of that initial reality of mine, let me take off this journey with you with some basic descriptions and explanations of autism before I proceed any further. This is to ensure that my readers are able to appreciate what the elements of mystery, confusion, anxiety and so forth captured in my stories hereunder really are. That particular context will also help to get a sense of the needs of persons living with autism.

The word **autism** is derived from the Greek word *autos* (meaning "self"") as used in *autonomous*. William Stillman, a renowned author on Autism and Asperger's Syndrome, in his book **The Autism Answerbook(2007)** says autism has been used to describe individuals who appear to be self-contained or who exist in their own little world, an inner realm seemingly set apart from others. By way of definition, Stillman thinks "these individuals have been clinically characterized as intentionally withdrawn and lacking in social reciprocity due to their communication difficulties or seeming disregard for social norms, as demonstrated through repetitive actions such as repeated hand flapping or infinitely spinning the wheel of a toy truck instead of rolling the truck along on all four tires".

The British National Autistic Society defines autism as a lifelong developmental disability which affects how people communicate and interact with the world. Physiologically, autism is considered as a common neurological anomaly that may preclude the body from properly receiving signals transmitted by the brain, resulting in misfires and disconnects. Likewise, the American Psychiatric Association defines the autism spectrum as consisting of five variations collectively called persuasive developmental disorders, and these are autistic disorder, Asperger's disorder, Rett's disorder, childhood disintegrative, and persuasive developmental disorder.

Mansah Gaisie Barnes has also explained that "autism is a neural developmental disorder characterized by impaired social interaction and communication, and also restricted and repetitive behavior in people who have it. No one knows the exact cause of autism. It varies widely in its severity and symptoms, and because of this early signs may go unrecognized, especially in mildly affected children or when it is masked by more debilitating handicaps".

There are certain classic characteristics of autistic behavior that are easily observable. Many children with autism experience a delay in talking or do not develop speech at all. They also have challenges communicating through nonverbal gestures such as making eye contact, using appropriate facial expressions and body language. They often seem to prefer to play alone, and may have a very intense preoccupation with a certain item or toy. Generally, children with autism tend to engage in specific rituals or routines, and may become upset when disrupted. Where they make physical movements, they often limit themselves to particular postures, like constant rocking, flapping of hands, spinning the body and repeated twitching of the eyes.

There are two major manifestations of autism that makes it awful and often generates disaffection and resentfulness from neighbors and the public, especially where such people are unexposed or uneducated about the condition. These are meltdowns and shutdowns. A meltdown is a state where the autistic person feels completely overwhelmed by the current situation or circumstances around him or her, and therefore loses behavioral control. It can result in shouting, screaming, crying, or physical outbursts like kicking, biting and lashing out at the nearest person. Children with autism experience meltdowns a lot, and they and their parents get blamed or judged by members of the public for throwing meaningless tantrums. A shutdown, on the other hand is a less intense response to being overwhelmed. Children with autism may become passive, quiet and could even switch off. It makes them unresponsive to speech, signals, promptings and even become difficult to manage or nurture. This may persist longer than a meltdown and could affect the child's progress in learning formally.

Autism is typically diagnosed after age two, but it is not considered a disease like other childhood ailments. It is therefore not degenerative, and modern medicine does not yet have the knowledge or expertise to prevent it. There are several theories about the causes of autism. Some scientists believe it is genetic, but others also say it is triggered by environmental factors such as viruses. There are also social theories like when the father is middle aged at conception, overexposure of children to television screens, and exposure of pregnant mothers to toxic pollutants. A typical child with autism is usually very fit physically and without any impairment or infirmity. Autism is four to five times more common in males than in females. The reason for this is not yet known. According to paedeatric practitioners, there are early warning signs parents and guardians should look out for with regards to autism in children. They include but are not limited to the following behaviors by the child:

a) not responding to speech

b) playing alone

c) using gestures to indicate a need rather than spoken language

d) intense expressions of frustration, otherwise called tantrums

e) lack of direct eye contact from the child

f) interest in routines and repetitive actions

g) overboard fascination/fixation with a toy or a part of it to the exclusion of all others

h) lack of regard or understanding of personal safety

i) low sense of danger

j) acute reactions to sensory sensitivities such as sounds, tastes, textures, smells, bright lights and temperatures

k) loss of language or learned skills

l) acts of deafness

Families with a child with autism have to endure the challenges of the disorder, emotional distress, depression, chaos and frustration. Their finances get overstretched from excessive medical bills and feeding costs. They have to repeatedly replace home appliances destroyed by the child with autism. Children with autism often engage in throwing things, knocking down furniture, making holes in walls and even destroying their own toys very fast. Perhaps a bigger challenge is the fact that it is very difficult to find qualified and willing persons to take care of a child with autism. Paying good caregivers can also be a major cost item in the family budget in addition to high medical bills and feeding costs for their irregular diets.

From my personal experience, I can say quite emphatically that autism causes a lot of changes and disruptions to the lives of families and individuals. Raising and nurturing a child with autism, and for that matter anybody living with autism is very hard work. It demands a response or a call to emergency action by parents, siblings, neighbours and the medical community. It requires an understanding and a resolve to embrace the autistic person and systematically device comprehensive and meaningful ways of living with and nurturing him or her appropriately. Practitioners and special education professionals suggest that society should approach autism by presuming intellect in the person with autism, and interact with him or her with a belief in his or her competence as gently and respectfully as we would anyone else.

As a parent I believe that an additional good response to autism is to re-envision each individual with autism as possessing thought processes that are fully intact, such that

we engage them not as though they are impaired or having physical limitations. There is so much to be achieved with autistic persons and that calls for welcoming them, accepting their differences and creating their space for them within our societal settings. I believe my stories as told further on in this book would illustrate and reveal this fact, and also bring to the fore the beauty of their breakthroughs and successes. There are many stories of high achievers in the past who have in recent years been perceived to have been autistic, because researchers studied their behaviors and activity patterns after they passed on. Such persons include Temple Grandin, Vincent Van Gogh, Thomas Edison, Leonardo da Vinci and Charles Darwin. There are some others living today and achieving marvelous feats who are also believed to be autistic, diagnosed or otherwise. Persons like Stephen Wiltshire, the young British artist, must motivate our society to accept, encourage and empower persons with autism amongst us by making room for their inclusion in our homes, schools, workplaces, social spaces and holistic social life.

In these 12 Dates, my experiences were not only about the highs and lows of living with autism, nor the battles for acceptance and inclusion of my son in our regular societal life. I also recognized, in rather unusual, confusing and uncertain circumstances, the eternal fact that the Holy Spirit is present with us in every situation of our lives, and that we could hear from Him if we pause and listen for His word. My 12 Dates are not just about my challenging circumstances dealing with autism, but about the involvement of the Holy Spirit and His interest in our everyday life issues. It is telling the story of ordinary people in our society, people living the Christian life with the help of the Holy Spirit, people confused, frustrated, tired and yet hopeful of a stable future for their own. People focused on the promises of God and living by faith in the face of seemingly unchanging and somewhat impossible situations. It is the story of how my family has lived and learnt to listen from within our hearts to the voice of the Holy Spirit for years as He whispers every now and again words and messages that sound like the reassuring words of Jesus to the disciples in **Mark 6: 31,** saying, ***"Come aside by yourselves to a deserted place and rest a while" (NKJV).*** I have heard His still small voice in many situations. Those recounted in this book are the specifics where He spoke to direct, comfort, strengthen and reassure me about what is going on about autism in the world, the challenges it has brought to families like mine and how we could count on Him and the sufficiency of His grace. I can say my perspective is widening and my understanding is deepening as I continue to reflect on the things I have shared in this book. I think the Reverend Gregory Hotchkiss makes the point I am struggling to make very succinctly in his statement that:

"the Lord does not come to put His stamp of approval upon our views and conclusions about life and about Him and His mission. Rather, He comes and gently but ever firmly intrudes with His Word, and He says, 'Listen, it is not as you had thought".

Let me at this juncture bring in my very brief profile of the Holy Spirit, just so that my dates with Him as recounted in this book can be better understood and appreciated. Importantly, let me hasten to add that the subject of discussing the person, work and ministry of the Holy Spirit is way beyond the scope of this work and thus is not in the slightest of imaginations part of the intention and goal of this book. It is however my fervent hope that this brief profile would reveal to and educate my readers a bit on the influence and enablement of the Holy Spirit in the lives of Christian believers such that they would receive Him, obey Him and participate in His interventions in their personal lives. This is important, because there is a very practical side of the advent of the Holy Spirit in the heart of mankind, by which He allows men and women to exercise the same authority with which Jesus overcame everyone of the limitations of mortality and trappings of sin in this world.

I begin by saying that the HOLY SPIRIT is a divine person, one of the three persons of the Triune God. He is called the Spirit of God, Spirit of the Lord, Spirit of Jesus and the Spirit of Truth. We know He is present with us and in our everyday lives from what the Bible says about Him. **Genesis 1:2** says *"the earth was without form and void, and darkness was on the face of the deep. And the Spirit of God was hovering over the face of the waters".*

From **Psalm 33:6,** we know that *"by the word of the Lord the heavens were made, and all the host of them by the Breath of His mouth."* **Job 33:4** also informs us that *"The Spirit of God has made me, and the Breath of the Almighty gives me life".* Again, from **Luke 1:35** we learn from Mary's experience thus, *"And the angel answered and said to her, "The Holy Spirit will come upon you, and the power of the Highest will overshadow you, therefore also, that Holy One who is to be born will be called the Son of God"*

His personality is further revealed to us in the Bible as follows; He is Eternal *(Hebrews 9:14), Omnipresent (Psalm 139:7-10), Omniscient (1 Corinthians 2:10-11), Almighty (Luke 1:35-37) and Holy (Romans 1:4).*

In the lives of true believers, He manifests in His fruit (**Galatians 5:22-24, Romans 8:23**) as well as by His gifts (**1 Corinthians 12:3-11, Exodus 31:3**). He baptizes us (**Acts 2:17-18,38**) and (**1 Corinthians 12:13**). Generally, He indwells our persons and everyday lives by transforming us (**1Corinthians 3:16, Ephesians 5:18, John 14:16-17**), and actually illuminates our lives with His understanding (**John 16:13-14**). Because He loves us so much, He has and will forever avail Himself to us as teacher, helper and comforter. This is very evident in what He tells us in His word (**John 14:26**).

Practically, many Christians have experienced the Holy Spirit in diverse ways. In fact Paul said quite forthrightly that *"each is given the manifestation of the Spirit for the common good".* He manifests in different ways in the circumstances of our lives in order to guide us. My reading of the book of Nehemiah points me to one such manifestation. Nehemiah talks about "that burden in his heart to see the walls of Jerusalem rebuilt and the temple restored".

Nehemiah 2:12 & 18 read as follows *"then I rose in the night, I and a few men with me. I told no one what God had put in my heart to do at Jerusalem, nor was there any animal with me, except the one on which I rode. And I told them of the hand of God which had been good upon me, and also of the king's words that he had spoken to me. So they said, 'Let us rise up and build'. Then they set their hands to this good work".*

We all sometimes feel burdened about something or someone and their situation, so much so that we assume a duty to pray and care for them. That is the Holy Spirit at work in us. The Apostle Paul shares his experiences with the Holy Spirit for our benefit. For example in **Acts 17** he tells us how he was provoked in his spirit and received a direction and ambition to preach to the Gentiles. In like manner, in our everyday lives the Holy Spirit uses our joys, pains, hardships, achievements, successes and failures to relate to us and to make His ways and purposes known. It is a blessing when we know and understand this, because we are then able to obey and cooperate with Him for marvelous outcomes in this life.

Some personal encounters and testimonies of other believers have taught me quite a number of things about how the Holy Spirit engages us. The Spirit of God has been speaking since creation. His purpose is to get us listening to and obeying God. Throughout the scriptures, we see Him speaking to people. From addressing their personal fears to meeting their destined needs, and from the rise and fall of nations, kingdoms and empires, the Holy Spirit has been speaking. He desires that we speak to Him, expecting that He will respond in His unique ways. Every believer needs to believe that He is, and then we can start a relationship and regular conversations with Him. Once a believer seeks Him with a searching heart, He will show up in one way or the other, and eventually make Himself well known to us.

As Chris Tiegreen puts it, "many believers are uncomfortable with the reality of the Holy Spirit, but Jesus made His presence foundational to the life of discipleship. We can only become disciples living the faith when the

Holy Spirit behind the biblical words writes them on our hearts and lives them through us. He spoke to Paul, John, Peter and others, and He still speaks". In fact F W Faber is reputed to have remarked that there is hardly ever a complete silence in our soul. God is whispering to us from very nearby circumstances all the time.

The Holy Spirit is a spiritual person, and He has a spiritual voice which we can learn to recognize. This is neither a science nor an art, supposedly reserved for prophets and pastors, theologians and spiritual leaders alone. It is for all the children of God, the people God created who have received Him as Lord out of their personal free will. For such people, their hearts and ears are spiritually open to the voice of the Holy Spirit and they hear Him speak to them. We hear the Holy Spirit in various ways, and He often tailors the message to fit our personalities and postures. Because the Holy Spirit is creative, His presence, voice and other manifestations are all mediums by which he engages us. He creatively uses words, pictures, emotions, events, miracles, wonders and so forth to get our attention and also to confirm His purposes.

As humans we are impure, and yet we have to relate with absolute purity. We therefore require a distilling discipline and attitude to recognize Him correctly. We can easily end up seeing what we want to see or hearing what we wish to hear. We can actually get it all wrong, and that is why every word, vision or feeling He gives us is made subject to testing. The Holy Spirit Himself says we should test the authenticity of His voice by checking if the Bible has said what we hear, or that He has confirmed it by His witnesses (apostles in our fold) or that He has provided supernatural signs to indicate His presence.

The Holy Spirit manifests when we respond in faith to His word. That is how He builds us up, just like we also feed our children to grow them up. When we respond in faith, He increases our faith to make us more like Him, and then He fulfills our purpose on earth by bearing His fruit in us.

The Holy Spirit is available to all believers in our everyday lives. We often mistakingly think that the Holy Spirit is in Heaven minding His business, and if only we prayed and waited long enough in fastings would He visit us and do a few miracles to show us His power. But the truth is, as Sarah Swindoll puts it, the Holy Spirit is accessible to us. He is already at work, and one simply needs to receive Him and participate in what He is doing. We must simply enter into His guidance and go where He leads, and receive what He has to offer us, and not wait for Him to come on a special day to us. The Holy Spirit is not far away in Heaven. He is invisibly around the believer all the time (John 14:17).

David Hernandez teaches us from his experience of the baptism of the Holy Spirit that one proof of the Holy Spirit in one's life is that godly character has been formed in him/her. He explains that the signs of the power of the Holy Spirit is not necessarily proof, because people can fake that power, and Satan actually enables them to do that. But the presence of the Holy Spirit in one's life shows in the character they live by, as described in **Galatians 5:22-23**, which states that *"the fruit of the Spirit is love, joy, peace, long-suffering, kindness, goodness, faithfulness, gentleness, self-control."* So speaking in tongues for instance is not the only proof of the Holy Spirit's presence in a man. The emphatic proof , as stated in **1 John 2:27** is that we can receive the Holy Spirit, and when we do, He lives within us and teaches us the truth and enables us to have fellowship with Him. This is how and why we can individually know when the Holy Spirit speaks in our everyday situations, when He advises us, when He stops us, when He rebukes us, when He encourages us and when He gives us hope and peace, even in chaotic situations.

The Holy Spirit is all powerful and can dramatically seize man's attention. He can actually speak compulsively to man like He did with Saul on the road to Damascus, and with Mary about her conception of the Saviour. He also does reveal amazing and compelling things in silence, like He did with Zacharias (Luke 1:59-68) and with Simeon in the temple (Luke 2:25-32). Yet He sometimes chooses to deal gently with us individually, and even waits patiently for us to give Him attention.

One major objective of this book is to help my readers notice and understand that there are signs, moments, coincidences, encounters and the like that simply mean that the Holy Spirit has shown up in our lives and is trying to get our attention. Particularly, when believers feel overwhelmed by circumstances and seem to have lost control of things looking at the way they had planned them, they get distracted and sometimes become stubborn such that they refuse to hear from God. Ironically, and interestingly, I have seen that the Holy Spirit remains with us through such times just so He can help us. I share just seven signs and moments here hoping that it would make us more alert and responsive to the Holy Spirit in our individual lives.

First of all, the Holy Spirit says some things repeatedly to us. There are times when we hear the same word of scripture repeated several times within a short period. Sometimes in one day or week or month, we may hear the same word of instruction in a sermon, song, devotional and the like from different people and at different places. The Holy Spirit is consistent when He is instructing us. In such moments, believers realize they have a heaviness of heart that persists until they obey the Holy Spirit. This is different from when you have a thought repeatedly come to mind or show up in your dreams.

Secondly, the Holy Spirit uses other people to confirm His word. I have seen this in the story of Samuel and Eli in the book of 1 Samuel in the Bible. But I see a more precise and exact scenario in **Acts 10:1-20**. The Holy Spirit clearly spoke to Cornelius and Peter, connecting and confirming His word of instruction. A careful reading of this chapter reveals about the Holy Spirit, how deliberate and progressive He is. Acts 10:15 reads *"and a voice spoke to him again the second time, 'What God has cleansed you* *must not call common'. This was done three times. And the object was taken up into heaven again".* Acts 10:19-20 also state *"while Peter thought about the vision, the Spirit said to him, Behold, three men are seeking you. Arise therefore, go down with them, doubting nothing, for I have sent them".* These verses illustrate that the Holy Spirit is both consistent and confirming of His word and intentions. He is very decisive about us and follows through with His purposes for us, using anybody and everything to get us to obey His promptings.

A third sign of the Holy Spirit relating with us as believers is His conviction when we have ignored or disobeyed Him. I have seen and appreciated this so very personally that sometimes I think James 4:17 is written for me alone. It reads *'therefore to him who knows to do good and does not do it, to him it is sin".* The Holy Spirit is forgiving by nature, and He brings conviction into our hearts to enable Him save us and continue to live in us. When we respond in obedience to His conviction, He then enables us to live with supernatural success.

The Holy Spirit also allows chaos in our lives, even up to the level of shipwreck. I see this when I read and reflect on the story and experiences of Jonah. **Jonah 1:14** profoundly says it all. It reads as follows, *"therefore they cried out to the Lord and said, 'we pray, O Lord, please do not let us perish for this man's life', and do not charge us with innocent blood, for You, O Lord, have done as it pleased You".* What is striking is that the sailors, being unbelievers, now prayed to the God of Jonah (Jehovah) revealing how they believed He (Holy Spirit) had sent the storm upon Jonah for His own good reasons. The Holy Spirit uses even the chaos in our lives. The destiny and life threatening misfortunes, temptations, accidents, betrayals, even our mistakes and so forth can all be used by Him to make us succeed, if only we would turn around and live in obedience to Him. Personally, when I reflect on Jonah 1:14 and Acts 27:9-15 together, I am able to believe completely what **Romans 8:28** says, that *"and we know that all things work together for good to those who love God, to those who are the called according to His purpose"*. I sincerely call on all believers to maintain a faith in this word, that God has actually said all things will eventually work together for our good. Let this faith encourage you to love God and face life and all of its issues daily, beholding yourself as a winner, and not a loser.

The fifth sign I wish to point to is that the Holy Spirit gives us inner peace. This peace is part of the fruit of the Holy Spirit which He bears in the lives of believers. He brings this peace when we are struggling with unexpected changes in our life situations. He also does this when we are contemplating major decisions. We can benefit from this when we make time to pray and seek the voice of God before we make very important decisions. When we fail to wait and listen out for the voice of the Holy Spirit, we sometimes make decisions which turn out bad. But interestingly, just thereafter our own inner voice makes us convinced that we were prompted not to do what we just did or decided. We must listen, and we will hear from Him.

Again, the Holy Spirit points us to the written word (logos) in the Bible in a way that appropriately brings the guidance and direction in such word to align with our circumstances. When we pay attention to the eternal truth and set standards in the Bible, we are able to tell when He leads us to read, or reminds us of the scriptures we know to help us understand and apply same to situations that demand life transforming decisions from us. A classic example of this is seen in Matthew 4:1-11 where the Lord Jesus relied on the written word to overcome and defeat the devil when he came against Him in his three-fold temptation. The Holy Spirit was with Him as He spoke to the devil with characteristic accuracy and power to disable and defeat him with the written word.

The sign number seven which I can share here is that the Holy Spirit comes to reveal deep secrets and hidden truths. He reveals coming events which no humans are able to foretell. We see this in the experiences of men like Moses at the burning bush, Saul on the road to Damascus, Jacob at Bethel, and Abraham at Mount Moriah.

Furthermore, the Bible reveals the person, the nature and the presence of the Holy Spirit to us by the use of certain symbols. A few of these are discussed here to drive home the point that we can know, perceive and identify the Holy Spirit personally. This is because He has graciously given us such privilege and knowledge. In Genesis 2:7, we learn that God breathed upon Adam the breath of life, making him a living being. This breath is the Holy Spirit. We can be confident in this knowledge because Job for instance identified with Him succinctly when he says in Job 32:8 that "*but there is a spirit in man, and the inspiration of the Almighty giveth them understanding.*" This symbol of the breath actually means the Holy Spirit is invisible and can relate with us unexpectedly.

The Holy Spirit is also symbolized as a dove (Luke 3:22). This is meant to illustrate His character, which He imbues within us when we receive Him. So we can tell when we have received Him, because He comes to cultivate in us gentleness, tenderness and purity.

Another symbol of the Holy Spirit is oil, which functions as unction and anointing (Luke 4:18). The Holy Spirit actually gives us understanding of heavenly truths, and enables us to worship in spirit and in truth as we are instructed in John 16:4 and Philippians 3:3.

The Holy Spirit is again symbolized with fire, which demonstrates His presence as seen in Acts 2:3-4, and taught by John in Luke 3:16-17 and Matthew 3:11-12. This illustrates His cleansing power through the conviction He brings into our hearts.

Jesus characteristically used the image of living water to identify the Holy Spirit. He told the Samaritan woman that the Holy Spirit, being living water, would live in the person who receives Him (John 4:14). This symbol shows the presence of the Spirit in our hearts which refreshes us and quenches our thirst. He brings us life when desolation and death threaten us. According to Charles Spurgeon, "the Holy Spirit seals us and makes us understand Him as our solemn guarantee of the salvation of God. We can rely on Him and be filled with joy at the thought of the moment when we shall be effectively filled unto all the fullness of God"

Let me conclude my brief profile of the Holy Spirit by sharing what Apostle Paul wrote to the church in Ephesus regarding the mission of the Holy Spirit in revealing to us the mystery, purpose and appreciation of Jesus Christ and godliness in Him. **Ephesians 3:3-21** reads as follows:

"How that by revelation He made known to me the mystery (as I have briefly written already, by which when you read you may understand my knowledge in the mystery of Christ), Which in other ages was not made known to the sons of men, as it has been revealed by the Spirit to His holy apostles and prophets.

That the Gentiles should be fellow heirs of the same body, and partakers of His promise in Christ through the gospel, of which I became a minister according to the gift of the grace of God given to me by the effective working of His power.

To me, whom am less than the least of all the saints, this grace was given, that I should preach among the Gentiles the unsearchable riches of Christ,

And to make all see what is the fellowship of the mystery which from the beginning of the ages has been hidden in God who created all things through Jesus Christ,

To the intent that now the manifold wisdom of God might be made known by the church to the principalities and powers in the heavenly places, according to the eternal purpose which He accomplished in Christ Jesus our Lord,

In whom we have boldness and access with confidence through faith in Him. Therefore I ask that you do not lose heart at my tribulations for you, which is your glory.

For this reason I bow my knees to the Father of our Lord Jesus Christ, from whom the whole family in heaven and earth is named, that He would grant you, according to the riches of His glory, to be strengthened with might through His Spirit in the inner man,

That Christ may dwell in your hearts through faith, that you being rooted and grounded in love, may be able to comprehend with all the saints what is the width and length and depth and height,

To know the love of Christ which passes knowledge, that you may be filled with all the fullness of God

NOW to Him who is able to do exceedingly abundantly above all that we ask or think, according to the power that works in us, to Him be glory in the church by Christ Jesus to all generations, forever and ever. Amen."

My goal in putting this together is to equip readers with knowledge to facilitate their choices and decisions, to listen quietly to one's inner voice in moments of confusion, frustration, anxiety and stress. It is to emphasize particularly to Christian believers the need to dwell on one's intimate knowledge and relationship with the Holy Spirit to receive strength, wisdom and hope to continue pursuing the good, regardless of the mounting disruptions in life. It is also to encourage everybody, especially people who have not believed and received the Lord Jesus Christ as personal savior, to read carefully the Word of God(Bible). This is because as **Deuteronomy 30:11-14** says, the commandment of God to us in our everyday and daily lives is not mysterious nor far away from us, but very near to us, in our own confessions of mouth and also in our hearts.

We must be looking out for the instances where humans who found themselves dealing with seemingly impossible and overwhelming situations in their everyday pursuits suddenly encountered the divine person of Jesus Christ, and received a new sense of purpose and strength to fight the good fight for life in Him. This is not an abstraction as some continue to think. It is the reality of life which is very clearly shown us in the gospel of Luke. The account in **Luke 24:13-27** presents a picture of a fleeting encounter with the Lord by men in their ordinary day activities without knowing so, and the Lord took advantage of that encounter to expound to them things concerning Himself in the scriptures and prophets.

Before concluding this introduction and invitation to you to enjoy reading my memoir, I wish to emphasize again that the Bible gives us many clear promises that the Lord (Holy Spirit) leads us and will always lead us. *Psalm 32:8 assures us as God tells us that He will guide us;*

"I will instruct you and teach you in the way you should go, I will guide you with My eye". In like manner, we are assured of the voice and satisfaction of God in the book of Isaiah. *"Your ears shall hear a word behind you, saying, 'This is the way, walk in it', whenever you turn to the right hand or whenever you turn to the left"* **(Isaiah 30:21)**. *"The Lord will guide you continually, and satisfy your soul in drought, and strengthen your bones; You shall be like a watered garden, and like a spring of water, whose waters do not fail"* **(Isaiah 58:11)**

It is my hope and expectation that as you read my stories herein, you would get exposed to and probably grow familiar with the different ways the Holy Spirit leads us. My remote mentor, the vintage Corrie ten Boom expatiated on this when she said that ***"the Lord leads us through His Word, through feelings and through circumstances, and mostly through all three together. It is such a wonderful experience when the Lord speaks through our feelings and our thinking when we pray and listen to the Lord. The prayer becomes then a conversation from both sides. We on our side must also learn to expect that the Lord acts according to His promises and lead us on His way."***

When we have learned these from the word and internalized them, we would be enabled to remember and see with the eyes of hope, and also receive the faith with which we would be able to hear from the Holy Spirit. I can say without a doubt, that when one hears from the Holy Spirit in a moment of distress and brokenness, a new strength in every form necessary becomes available, and that is the only real thing that overcomes.

Enjoy reading, and do well to take away with you hope and the joy of the Lord as your strength for life's battles.

LONELY NIGHTS

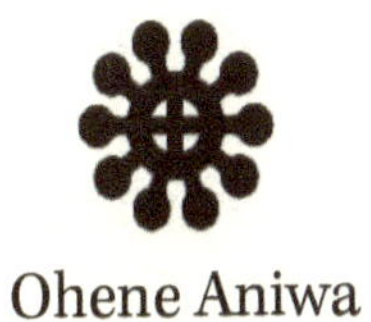

Ohene Aniwa

I dedicate this chapter to my dear son Yooku Sompa, whose challenging life with autism has substantially impacted my personal life, my interests and outlook to human relationships, and eventually birthed this idea of a book in me.

Yooku was born in the year 2002. He had a lovely childhood, growing through the first year milestones and started pre-school soon after age two. Sometime at age three he begun to lose his speech of few words which he was noted for repeating happily to us. Before long, alarm bells were sounded to us by his school care-givers, pediatrician and our parents. They had made closer and deeper observations beyond what Sheila and I as his parents had complained about to them regarding Yooku not speaking anymore. We gave ourselves the task of giving him a bit more time to come back to his sweet self from the "supposed new habits" of keeping to himself, lining up his toys, covering his ears once the lights were turned on, sitting in one corner of the family room all alone, avoiding eye contact with us, repeating some unusual noises intermittently and losing interest in virtually everything. Suddenly, he was disinterested in everybody's attention. So we compared notes, continued observing, and compared notes again and again for about three months. One day when we visited the pediatrician, he said something that would probably never leave my memory again. "The question of autism crosses my mind", he said. So we went on to seek help. Yooku was assessed and diagnosed as a child on the autism spectrum. We were counseled and started off on the journey of our new life of living with autism.

This chapter is about nights from that day and how lonely some of them have been ever since. But more importantly it is about a few of those nights when out of the loneliness and strife the Holy Spirit moved me to reconciliation and communion with Himself. When Yooku was between three and five years of age, many nights were sleepless for me. This was not like the familiar ones that parents know about when, due to sickness, pain or some uneasiness and discomfort the child cannot sleep and hence parents do not sleep. The routine was that Yooku would either stay awake moving around the rooms in the home, sit with his toys or sometimes just sit on his bed with crossed legs, rather than lie down. There were nights of continuous humming, clapping or laughing loudly and so forth. But I saw all such behaviors as the new normal and though annoying, we could handle them without much stress. There were also those nights when Yooku would cry, sob, moan and practically hold on to me or his mum and lie down in his pain, hoping to fall asleep. I dare say even a baby could tell in those days how deep Yooku's sorrows were as a child. It was obvious something was eating him up and yet he could not voice it out.

The disturbing new night situation which really brought

on my feeling of loneliness was when I began to observe after we had obtained a prescription for sleeping pills to help his night sleep, that he would only sleep for about two hours and then wake up. I used to go to check on him alone during the quiet night hours to be sure he was safely asleep, and I found out that he was often sitting up with crossed legs and chin in his palms, looking pensively at the blank wall beside the bed. I was always troubled to behold that sight, because I could not imagine what on earth a little child like him could be thinking about so deeply as he seemed to be. He did not look sick, restless or as if suffering some discomfort. He simply looked pensive and deep in thought. I often sat near him and rocked his back for some time till we would both fall asleep. I had no responses or gestures of agreement from him when I sought to pray with him. It was always a moment of brokenness for me, and I was quite unwilling to share that experience with anybody. It was a while before I could tell even my wife about it. A psychological battle had started in me, and I could not ward it off. I would sometimes go to the office worn out and visibly troubled. I often had a lot on my mind and could not concentrate on any work I was supposed to do. My mind would roam and roam about the question of what my life would be now with this autism that appeared so difficult to understand.

One night, I went to sit by Yooku on his bed again. I decided to just sit still and only mimic whatever he would do. A few minutes later I started singing a hymn to him. I sang very softly Keith Green's oldie, Oh Lord, You're Beautiful. Yooku's reaction was amazing. He seemed to hum along but only for the first line, and waited for me to finish the verse. I sang a second and third time, and then he stretched out and lay down. I continued singing, and on the seventh time he closed his eyes and fell asleep. I thanked God and went to my room after about twenty minutes. This became a new routine for me. But one day Yooku wouldn't sleep while I was singing, so I slept on his bed and kept singing till I fell asleep myself. When I woke up he was sleeping soundly. I made the lyrical plea of the song part of my prayer for him, and still say that prayer for him all these years. This is what it says:

1. Oh Lord, You're beautiful
Your face is all I seek
For when Your eyes are on this child
Your grace abounds to me.
Oh Lord, You're beautiful
Your face is all I seek
For when Your eyes are on this child
Your grace abounds to me.
I wanna take Your word and shine it all around
But first help me to just live it Lord
And when I'm doing well

Help me to never seek a crown
For my reward is giving glory to You.

2. Oh Lord please light the fire
That once burnt bright and clear
Replace the lamp of my first love
That burns with holy fear.
I wanna take Your word
And shine it all around
But first help me to just live it Lord
And when I'm doing well
Help me to never seek a crown
For my reward is giving glory to You.

3. Oh Lord You're beautiful
Your face is all I seek
For when Your eyes are on this child
Your grace abounds to me.

Thus the nights of singing for him to sleep continued for

months. There were days and seasons when the sleep would still not be long enough, and one had to manage with walking around the living room or sitting by and watching him through the night hours. There was a day I picked him up from school, and on our way home he fell asleep, snoring quite loudly. I muttered to myself, that he might end up not sleeping at night. Then I thought also that the miracle song might just not work that night. Just at that moment I heard the voice of the Holy Spirit within me say, **"I grant sleep to those I love. It is my gift and reward. It is not in singing a song"**. It was a sobering moment and experience for me. Thank God for repentance. All alone and in the quiet of my heart, I asked His forgiveness and prayed that I would recognize His work in our lives as a family and be grateful. I kept thinking about that word all the way home, and it became clearer to me that God watches over us. Some scriptures I had read and seen in the Bible about God watching over us, and how He gives us sleep and rest from our toils came to my mind. I remember I pondered over verses like the following:

"It is vain for you to rise up early, to sit up late, to eat the bread of sorrows, for so He gives His beloved sleep. Behold, children are a heritage from the Lord, the fruit of the womb is a reward. Like arrows in the hand of a warrior, so are the children of one's youth." **Psalm 127:2-4.**

"The Lord looks from heaven, He sees all the sons of men. From the place of His dwelling He looks on all the inhabitants of the earth". **Psalm 33:13-14**

"Behold, He who keeps Israel shall neither slumber nor sleep. The Lord is your keeper, The Lord is your shade at your right hand". **Psalm 121:4-5**

"He will fulfill the desire of those who fear Him, He also will hear their cry and save them. The Lord preserves all who love Him, but all the wicked He will destroy". **Psalm 145:19-20.**

It then dawned on me that my son needed to have his own view and understanding of the God who loves him and grants him the blessings of sleep, rest and preservation.

I remember I prayed that God Himself would give him as a little child that love for Him as a friend, and think about Him sometimes. When we got home, my mind was preoccupied with what we could possibly do to put a picture of the Lord Jesus as an imprint on Yooku's mind. As bedtime stories are told to children to form in their infant minds and hearts a love for the Lord Jesus as Creator and Savior, I was looking for a means of achieving the same with my son, knowing very well that he was unable at that time to properly comprehend ideas and statements. But I was truly interested in doing that. So after dinner I asked my wife for another very nice song that tells about Jesus as a beautiful person whose love makes us safe. Guess what! She gave me the compact disc (CD) album of CeCe Winans with the song **"Jesus, You're Beautiful"**. She later shared with me when I explained to her what I had planned to do with that song, that she had been praying that somehow Yooku's mind would be conditioned and inspired by the scripture in **Psalm 63:6**, which reads, *"when I remember You on my bed, I meditate on You in the night watches"*.

This encouraged me further to work on getting the name

of the Lord Jesus on Yooku's mind. That weekend, I sat with my son alone and played the song over and over again, and we sang and hummed it happily to ourselves. Bit by bit the tune sunk into his head and he showed signs of enjoying it. I could tell it was having a soothing and calming effect on him, and we kept at it for quite a while. Soon, it had become part of the bedtime songs and the whole family used to sing it together for him to enjoy. He actually had a lovely way of repeating lines in the chorus, particularly 'so beautiful, so beautiful, so beautiful' and also Oh oh oh. The lyrics of the full song are as follows:

Jesus, bright as the morning star
Jesus, how can I tell You
How beautiful You are to me
Jesus, song that the angels sing
Jesus, dearer to my heart than anything.

Sweeter than spring time
Purer than sunshine
Ever my song will be
Jesus, You're beautiful to me.

Jesus bright as the morning star
Jesus how can I tell You
How beautiful You are to me
Jesus, song that the angel sing
Jesus, dearer to my heart than anything.

Sweeter then spring time
Purer than sunshine
Ever my song will be
Jesus, You're beautiful to me

Oh Lord You are so beautiful
Oh beautiful
So beautiful
So beautiful
Jesus, You're beautiful to me
Beautiful, beautiful, beautiful

Jesus, You're beautiful to me.
Morning star, Lord You are
Beautiful, Jesus, You're beautiful to me.
Oh, oh, oh, so beautiful

Sweeter than spring time
Purer than sunshine
Ever my song will be
Jesus, You're beautiful to me.

Jesus, how can I tell You
How beautiful You are to me
Jesus, song that the angels sing
Jesus, dearer to my heart than anything.

Sweeter than spring time
Purer than sunshine
Ever my song will be
Jesus, You're beautiful to me.

Jesus, bright as the morning star
Jesus, how can I tell You
How beautiful You are to me
Jesus, song that the angels sing
Jesus, dearer to my heart than anything

Sweeter than spring time
Purer than sunshine
Ever my song will be
Jesus, You're beautiful to me.

The challenge of sleeplessness, many thanks to God, has been largely overcome. Though we continue to administer prescribed night pills (sedatives), Yooku can sleep quite well and does not feel restless in the morning as was the situation in years gone by. We are grateful for the abundant mercies shown us. We are confident that Yooku can appreciate and comprehend it when we ask him to pray or sing praise to God, because he makes very consistent gestures and shows sobriety doing so. It remains our fervent prayer as a family that the good Lord would truly reveal Himself to him and enable him to live for Him, knowing Him as Lord and Savior of his life.

Romans 10:8-10 says: *"For salvation that comes from trusting Christ, which is what we preach, is already within easy reach of each of us; in fact it is near as our own hearts and mouths. For if you tell others with your own mouth that Jesus Christ is your Lord and believe in your own heart that God has raised Him from the dead, you will be saved. For it is by believing in his heart that a man becomes right with God; and with his mouth he tells others of his faith, confirming his salvation"* (NIV).

We cannot confirm what Yooku has said with his mouth and believed in his heart as he has not been able to confess (speak) to us his faith in the Lord. But we dwell on our faith and trust Christ for His salvation. We have received answers to our prayer for him regarding many things and specific challenges of his life, and so we continue to thank God for his salvation.

BROKEN HEARTS

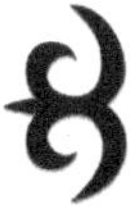

Akoko Nan Tia Ba

I pay my tribute for this chapter is to Michael Owusu Ansah and his dear wife Phyllis. Michael and Phyllis are leaders of the Children's Department in my church, and are wonderful servants of God who love children in an amazing way. I thank Michael and Phyllis very much for their love for the children of God, and for the many sacrifices they continue to make for people like my family and I. I truly thank God for their lives and pray they remain blessed.

My heart has been broken many times since coming into the experiential world of living with autism. In this chapter I have chosen to share a combination of three memorable encounters that I refer to for consolation and inspiration. The first was when I realized my son could not cry nor shed tears normally to express his pain or grief. I usually help him with his bath and body care routines in the morning and get him ready for school or any outing for the day. This could often get clumsy, because there are times when he just won't cooperate because he feels different, or unwilling to brush his teeth, take a bath and so forth. Sometimes one has to wait so long for him, or be tough to get him to hurry through the process in order not to be so late for regular schedules. In one particular week, he was very reluctant to brush his teeth, and took to spitting the tooth paste out whenever I tried helping him with it. He was clearly and consistently resisting my efforts to get the brush into his mouth. Out of frustration, he reacted by biting me. Four times in that week I had been bitten. Naturally I also became frustrated and confused. I actually thought he was trying to form another habit, and I did not want that as another autistic practice. How wrong I was. Yooku had bitten his tongue and was in pain. Being non-verbal, he could not express it, and my impatience made me fail to observe and inspect his mouth for any challenge he was having at the time. I just rushed him with it for us to go to school. One particular morning, I failed to read his sign language signal attempting to say "I'm sorry, I'm sorry, I'm sorry". He looked so sorrowfully at my face, went on his knees and held my foot. His eyes were red but had no tears. Everything in his demeanor told me he was weeping within him for my mercy on him, and yet I had failed to notice his plea. Then suddenly, I thought I heard the voice of my wife, who had already left the house about twenty minutes earlier, scream out to me saying, **"Leave my child alone, he is wounded. He is not being stubborn."** I looked around and she was not there. I ran to the gate, she wasn't there. On getting back to handle my son, it occurred to me that I had heard from my inner voice. I was being prompted and instructed by the Holy Spirit. How did I know that? Two things happened. First, I felt his grief instantly and lifted him up saying "I'm sorry,

Yooku". Second, I asked him, "Do you have a sore?" He took my hand into his foamy mouth and I could feel and see it right there. I had to apply lime-rub and chemical mouthwash for him, bathe him and feed him and then we got ready for school.

My heartbreak resulted from the fact that I could on that occasion cry out my regret for failing to understand and feel his pain, but he could not cry out his pain nor his sorrow over my shortcoming in that instance as his father and carer. I felt completely guilty, and it was a heavy grief for me because I truly love my son. My consolation has been that the forgiving Holy Spirit who wipes away all tears assures us all in His word that He does not hold such against us. He has empowered me with much more patience and understanding for my son, who is also His child. I have only recently learnt from one parent on one of the parents' networks I belong to, that the safest way to avoid emotional pain to these guys is to hug them and rub their back. Trust me it is working for us. I have also learnt that the inability to cry and shed tears is not unique to my son. This is all confusing and bothersome to me, knowing how soothing and cleansing tear-drops can be to a grieving person.

Autism is notorious for changing lives. One of the ways this comes about is that families have to become selective about places to go to and events to attend. For my family, attending worship service in church on Sundays is a religious routine we hold in very high esteem. Autism's impact started changing our Sunday life too, and that brought about the second memorable experience of broken hearts selected for this chapter. When Siisi, my second son turned five, he used to attend the same class with Yooku for Sunday school in church even though they are almost three years apart. Siisi would tell me about the challenges Yooku had fitting into the class because there was no dedicated carer assigned to him. He sometimes told me how Yooku could become disruptive of the teaching process, would harass a particular child, or hit the teachers, or bite himself and scream, or scatter the toys and teaching tools when all the children were seated and so forth. Siisi was obviously sad about this situation, and hence was not as excited about going to church as he had been before anymore. I consoled him and decided I would join them in their class and sit with Yooku at the back of the class to control him, so the children could enjoy their classes without the disruptions. This worked well but for only three weeks, because the leaders of the Children's Department had noticed me and would not approve of my being there for my son's sake. I was advised to stop "invading" the children's service because they could manage my son. I had to oblige and obey, but that created a new challenge. The next Sunday when I told Siisi I was not joining them again in their class at Sunday school, he was heartbroken and lost all enthusiasm about going to church. It was then that he told me how unhappy he had been and how he wanted to continue to be in the class with Yooku without me. He said some of the children were not friendly and shunned him because of Yooku's challenges. He was sad because he felt some people did not love his brother. I had to console him and explain to him that those children did not understand Yooku's challenges and so they needed time to learn to accept and love him as he did. Siisi was confused about this and cried for a while on our way to church. After church he said emphatically that he didn't want to go to that class again. This was sad for me, because autism was beginning to impact our beautiful family life on Sunday too, and was actually confusing my Siisi as to acceptance of him and his brother in church. This certainly left me heart broken.

We skipped two Sundays and went back to church on the third. Yooku had a massive meltdown just before the close of the service. He went "bunkers", totally out of control: hitting, biting, kicking, ripping shirts, pulling hairs, throwing things and the like. He was taken to an empty classroom and was battling with four of the teachers. Michael Owusu Ansah called me out and came running to the portal of the auditorium to get me to come to help my son. When I got to the place, Yooku was drenched in sweat, looking scared and fierce, confused and very dirty. I grabbed him, hugged him tightly and sat with him on the bare floor. I got a bottle of water and poured it on his head. He was still hitting, so I got my belt off and bound his hands. He bit me on the left thumb, and smashed his chair against the wall. All this happened while the screaming and roaring continued. But he got tired, and slowed down a bit. We sat there on the floor for about ten minutes, and I continued rubbing and rocking him. The confused audience looked at us, and I wondered what we looked like and meant to them. I had mixed feelings of pain, loneliness and shame. Eventually, he became calm. Michael helped us to the car park, we got Yooku his first aid and went home. Many conversations with church folk followed this episode in the next few weeks. Michael and his team were instrumental so after our two weeks break from church, we were welcomed to a special classroom created for special needs children to have their own special worship service. This was a comforting breakthrough for which we are eternally grateful to God. I had many conversations with Michael thereafter; seminars and study sessions with the teachers and carers have followed and I have had opportunities to share ideas and knowledge. Our children have come a long way in learning to worship the Lord. I believe you agree that I have a good reason to pay tribute to Michael and Phyllis, and to say thank you to them for serving God's children the way they do, and to pray that they may be blessed so much by the Lord.

In June 2013 I drove into the Autism Centre one morning with my son, and had a short meeting with the Administrator. I had been away working a few weeks in China, and having returned home, I needed to touch base for an update on my son's programme in school. When I was leaving, a parent came in with her twin boys of about fifteen years. I observed how they got out of the car and started their different behaviours. Let me call them Kweku and Kuuku. These were hyperactive boys on the autism spectrum. One had a body spinning behavior, and the other was the finger-flapping and loud-laughing type. They were quite well built and of average height. It was very easy to tell that they had arrived, and the carers quickly came out to make way for them and to take them in to the sensory room to calm them down before they would be sent to their classroom. I was told they had been admitted just the week before, and came in every morning from home, about 40km away.

Grief-striken, I drove off to go pursue my day's business. Within 15 minutes I had to pull off the road and park nearby. Why? Because I was overwhelmed. Momentary thoughts of Kweku and Kuuku whom I had just seen and imaginations of what their family must be going through with them broke my heart with pain and sorrow. My fountain of tears had burst, my arms were frozen and I could not continue driving. I helped myself by parking for about half an hour to cry and heal. I asked God, **"Lord, isn't this too much for the family?"** Trust me, I got an instant answer from the Holy Spirit, soft but emphatic. He said, **"My grace is sufficient, and I am always around them"**. I can assure you, I didn't understand the real meaning of that word at that moment, I just cried a bit more, sat quietly for a while after cleaning up, got composed, and then went on my way. I still remember I did practically no meaningful work that day in the office, because my mind had shut down, and my heart was broken.

Knowing I was in trouble, I read some verses of scripture to help find myself. I settled on **Psalm 34:18** which reads *"The Lord is near to those who have a broken heart, and saves such as have a contrite spirit"*.

I meditated on it for most of the afternoon. This is my summary of the unction the Holy Spirit gave me that day about His word and this verse of scripture. First, He permits our hearts to get broken by certain events because He wants to be near us. The presence of the Holy Spirit with us is more important to Him than it is to us. He is here on earth for that primary purpose to be with us. Jesus said He was going away so the Holy Spirit would come (**John 14:16-18**). Secondly, the Holy Spirit is here with us implementing His own plan for us, and He uses our daily routines to instruct and direct us. Thirdly, the Holy Spirit comes to us to help us even before we go to Him or cry out for help. Fourthly, He is not only near us and with us. He actually dwells in us and actively works through us as long as we do not grieve Him. That is why we can hear Him speak to us from within us, and from around us when we learn to listen to His voice. Fifthly, He works for us. He teaches us the truth, and also brings to our remembrance all things. Sixthly, the Holy Spirit gives us peace, so that our hearts would not remain troubled. Seventhly, He loves us, and keeps us away from the troubling circumstances and demands of this world.

Playing back this unction over my experiences, from mistreating my son to the meltdown in church to imagining how the family of the twin boys (Kweku and Kuuku) may be suffering, I am convinced of and grateful for the presence of the Holy Spirit in my life. From this reality, I urge my readers to receive the Holy Spirit into their lives, learn to love Him and listen to His voice, and live this life with the enablement and empowerment He brings for our everyday walk on earth.

GUIDE HIS THOUGHTS, LORD

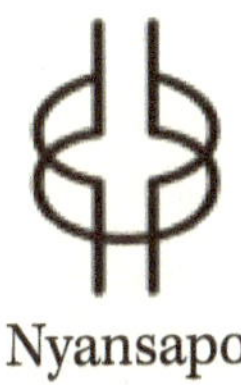

Nyansapo

This chapter's tribute goes to my dear father and senior friend, Richard Acquaah Harrison. Papa and Mama Muriel are a grand old couple and neighbors of my family at home. They are devoted Christians and lovers of chorale music. Papa loves me and so I visit him often at his home. When I do, we chat about various matters, from biblical issues, developments in the church, music, politics, education, family life and travels around the world, sometimes for hours. He has also been visiting my family in our home. Many thanks, Papa, for your friendship and encouragement all these years, particularly for what I am about sharing here on this journey.

I went home to Papa, Richard Acquaah Harrison, one evening at about 7pm. I had just taken my son home after a very difficult day, and I found Papa playing hymns on his piano. Because he is very friendly and accommodating, we got talking almost immediately. He could easily tell from my countenance that I was troubled, so he asked what the matter was. I told Papa about my day's events and the confusion I was dealing with as follows. We had brought in a new house-help only a few days earlier. That morning, the lady who I call Esi for purposes of this work spoke very ill words to my son while helping him get ready for school. My wife saw and heard her and naturally sought to correct and caution her about such improper behavior. Guess what, hell broke loose in my home. Esi wouldn't take anybody's correction. Rather, she gave my wife and I a dress down for being failures at correcting our son, and having seen him grow up without, in her view, any proper manners, and so we should not think she was going to allow him misbehave towards her. She was outrightly rude without any empathy in her reaction. In spite of our knowing that Esi was reacting in ignorance, we were both very hurt and discouraged. We instantly decided as couple that Esi was no good a helper in our home and thus needed to be sent away. My wife made arrangements for her to leave the same day.

Esi was the fifth person we could not live with within a period of about one year. Like the others, I had taken the trouble to explain to her the challenges with my son and the primary need for her to give him empathetic attention, self-care assistance and patient treatment with or without cooperation from him. I had tried to explain the behaviors of my son at home, his methods of communicating and seeking assistance for his basic needs and the difficulties he has which could easily put him in harm's way. The episode of that morning was evidence that my son living with autism may well be unsafe and subject to maltreatment even at home because our helpers may have misconceptions and bad attitudes towards him. I remembered how two visitors to our home virtually stopped their kids from playing with my son or staying close to him, and eventually decided to leave because they thought the autistic condition was infectious. One person told us to the face that "you better go and find a spiritual healer to save your son before you lose him to the demonic forces attacking him".

I recall another time where while eating with some friends at a birthday party, we got publicly insulted by two people for, in their words, failing to teach our child to behave himself, because in his excitement, he went round picking food from other peoples' plates around the table. These two persons felt so offended by our child's behaviour that they actually left the table for a new one far away from us. My good friend whose party we had attended then sought to intervene, but got told off too for bringing such an unruly family us ours to ruin their enjoyment that afternoon. On yet another occasion when I attended a public concert with him and sat in a far out corner of the theatre with him, his loud intermittent screams and continuous laughter as is usual of autistic children was probably strange to several people around us, so we observed them leave one by one to find new seats elsewhere in the theatre, ostensible to have their peace.

On the very day when Esi hurt our emotions so badly, a distant cousin of mine called me and plainly insulted me for talking about my son on radio. To her, my decision to grant an interview on a radio show in furtherance of public awareness about the condition and to advocate for better inclusion of children living with autism in our societal life was misguided. She advised me to stop doing that as it was only exposing my son and family to public ridicule and isolation, rather than education of the society, because in her view it was well known that such children are either bewitched or cursed, and would not be easily accepted by those who know this. This was all because just the week before I had a live broadcast interview on an Accra based radio station on the socialization of children living with autism as part of a month-long awareness campaign staged by the special school my son attended. Nothing I sought to say to explain to her how wrong her opinion was would be acceptable to her, so I just let her be, and told myself to forget about her insults. It was not easy to ward off that also from my mind.

Somehow, my son had picked up the negative posture and treatment he got at home that morning, so he was very withdrawn and morose in school. When I went to pick him up at close of day's business, his care giver asked questions about his demeanor for the day, pointing to a possible trigger from some unusual morning encounters. I shared a few words with her and off we went. The ride home was good, but my mind could not rest. When we got home, my wife was equally disturbed that we had to go through the tussle of finding and preparing another person to engage as house help again. Worse still she was concerned that the frequency of a new helper was bound to have its own negative impact on both our children's nurturing process and confidence. Yet it appeared we had no option in those circumstances because we were both employed with regular corporate organizations and had our schedules and working hours fairly fixed for us in those days. We thought a domestic helper was certainly necessary to keep the home in proper shape and on track. But the experiences were becoming not only discouraging and stressful, but a challenge to our patience, hope and confidence in the safety of our children with "these other people". I admitted to Papa that I was hurting and couldn't figure out what at all we had done to deserve such dejection.

Papa reached for his Bible, moved to sit next to me, and with his arm across my shoulders started praying for me. I remember vividly how he prayed saying, **"Lord guide his thoughts, and give his mind rest".** At that moment, I felt within my spirit (inner self- consciousness) as though certain objects up in the air and around me had just fallen and settled down. I could virtually feel stability and not chaos around me then. He continued praying for a few minutes and stopped, and we said Amen to that. He then opened his Bible and read to me this passage of scripture.

*"My brethren, count it all joy when you fall into various trials, knowing that the testing of your faith produces patience. But let patience have its perfect work, that you may be perfect and complete, lacking nothing. If any of you lack wisdom, let him ask of God, who gives to all liberally and without reproach, and it will be given to him. But let him ask in faith, with no doubting, for he who doubts is like a wave of the sea, driven and tossed by the wind." **James 1:2-6***

He gave me wise counsel and encouragement from this scripture. Being an old and very experienced man, he was familiar with the incidents I told him about and also understood such human behaviors well enough. Papa knew my son quite well then. He was present at his christening ceremony a few years earlier, and had his own way of handling and entertaining him as a child when he visited us, and so was convinced that he was not an untrained child. Being a widely travelled person, he had met several persons living with autism and had actually given me some documents on the condition and training facilities available for children with autism in Canada. He was positive and optimistic that my Yooku was capable of overcoming his challenges, and encouraged me to focus on that with faithful prayer. Explaining the import of the scripture he read to me, he said I needed to accept it that God's purpose for my son, my family and I was to overcome the problems by thinking correctly. He said we did not have to struggle for acceptance nor agree with people's perspectives about us and our situations when we knew they were wrong, and that the important thing is to always ask God for the wisdom to handle the challenges. We continued to chat for a while before I left for my home. To date, I do not know exactly why I decided to visit Papa that very night. One thing I know though is that I heard from the Holy Spirit that night through him, and I was greatly encouraged, strengthened and uplifted by that encounter. Frankly, having a child with autism sometimes leaves you helpless. You could be made to think you are at the mercy of others, and everyone may want to tell you how to take care of your child. That could be overwhelming and each family will have to deal with social alienation, segregation and emotional stress at one time or another. But I can also confidently say that the innocence of children living with autism is in itself an emphatic statement that they deserve acceptance, love and support. Their families deserve empathy, encouragement and assistance where possible.

In applying the counsel Papa gave me and reading further for wisdom from the Bible, I have learnt some more from the Holy Spirit to pray aright about confusing situations and trust God with optimism for His solutions at the right time. He has led me to several perspectives, statements and scriptures that have deepened my faith in Him and broadened my understanding of the role and place of disruptions in life. I share with you some of these nuggets.

"The best men are often molded out of faults". **Shakespeare.**

"The marvelous richness of human experience would lose something of rewarding joy if there were not limitations to overcome. The hilltop would not be half so wonderful if there were no dark valleys to traverse." **Helen Keller**

"Cultivate my heart Lord, so I may catch every word that falls from heaven, every syllable of encouragement, every sentence of rebuke, every paragraph of instruction, every page of warning. Help me to catch these words as the soft, fertile soil catches seeds" **Ken Gire.**

"Human felicity is produced not so much by great pieces of good fortune that seldom happen, as by little advantages that occur every day". **Benjamin Franklin**

"He who does not live in some degree for others hardly lives for himself" **Montaigue.**

"Lord, purge our eyes to see within the seed a tree, within the glowing egg a bird, within the shroud a butterfly, till taught by such we see beyond all creatures, Thee". **Christina Rossetti.**

*"Therefore we also, since we are surrounded by so great a cloud of witnesses, let us lay aside every weight, and the sin which so easily ensnares us, and let us run with endurance the race that is set before us, looking unto Jesus, the author and finisher of our faith, who for the joy that was set before Him endured the cross, despising the shame, and has sat down at the right hand of the throne of God." **Hebrews 12:1-2.***

*"In this you greatly rejoice, though now for a little while, if need be, you have been grieved by various trials, that the genuineness of your faith, being much more precious than gold that perishes though it is tested by fire, may be found to praise, honor, and glory at the revelation of Jesus Christ." **1 Peter 1:1-2.***

*"But sanctify the Lord God in your hearts, and always be ready to give a defence to everyone who asks you a reason for the hope that is in you, with meekness and fear, having a good conscience, that when they defame you as evildoers, those who revile your good conduct in Christ may be ashamed. For it is better , if it be the will of God, to suffer for doing good than for doing evil". **1 Peter 3:15-17.***

*"Though the fig tree may not blossom, nor fruit be on the vines; Though the labor of the olive may fail, and the fields yield no food; Though the flock may be cut off from the fold, and there be no herd in the stalls. Yet I will rejoice in the Lord, I will joy in the God of my salvation. The Lord God is my strength; He will make my feet like deer's feet, and He will make me walk on my high hills." **Habakkuk 3:17-19.***

KEEP HOPE ALIVE

Biribiwosoro

For this chapter, I pay tribute to my senior brother and good friend Charles Ofori Atta. Charles and I go back well over thirty good years. We met as mates in high school in the 1980s and have remained brothers in the faith, in ministry and in family life ever since. I thank Charles, for his friendship and helpful acts in times when I was almost desperate.

Charles and his heavily pregnant wife Cynthia had come to visit me at home one beautiful weekend when suddenly Cynthia said it was about her time to have the baby. Charles drove her off to the hospital, and a few hours later the lovely chubby Nana Yaw Adom was born. At this time I was not yet married, and so the birth of Nana Yaw gave me a great good feeling, and heightened in me a desire to have a son some time in the near future. Naturally, I have had a very special liking and love for Nana Yaw, and I have followed his growth and maturing process through the years.

One very beautiful afternoon, Charles came by my office. He had been to a meeting at the headquarters of one Department of State close by and stopped over for a brief visit. It was all joy when Charles shared the good news about Nana Yaw having gained admission to high school.

As usual, we spent the time chatting, and also prayed thanking God for graciously bringing our son that far in his young life. Our joy was so great also because Nana Yaw was going to the same noble school we had both attended in our youth. It was such a nostalgic moment for us.

When Charles was leaving we used the staircase down to the carpark. While walking he asked when I was to pick up Yooku after school that day. Rather unconsciously, I was sad, and momentarily wondered when and how Yooku's breakthrough would come, so he could also dream of a phase in his life when he could attain higher education and progress from there with hope of a good career in adult life. Charles noticed the change in my countenance and instantly demanded that we go back to my office. When we took our seats, he told me quite emphatically that he could tell I had become sorrowful because I was losing hope of the expectation that my Yooku would also be ready for senior high school one day. He went ahead and spoke very strongly and convincingly to me about what the devil could try to do to me and my family, just to cause us pain and a sense of rejection by our God. My friend was very fired up as he sought to encourage and inspire me to deal decisively with the thoughts, feelings and moments when bouts of dejection would hit me. He recounted times in the past when we had prayed so much for healing, for a breakthrough for my son to speak and also have a definite skill/talent manifested in him, so that we could concentrate his training and learning efforts on that to set him on a possible career path. I told him that frankly I sometimes felt not much change was coming through in Yooku's life, and yet he was growing very fast. I told Charles how tough it was sometimes for me, thinking about all the extra investments of money and time in him, the toils at night to keep him safe and rested, the many times I have been called by his school to come and take him home or for medical attention because he had become too stressed from a meltdown and so forth. My pain was that almost no change was coming in terms of a normalization in his behaviors and self-care in particular. I went on and on about how frustrating it was those days for me to continue praying for Yooku and keep hoping that his learning capabilities would improve. I was truly tempted to give up waiting and hoping for his speech, and the more crucial capability to learn formally as well as develop his innate skills through structured training and coaching. I had heard several times within my inner-man the intimidating voice of the devil, that Yooku would amount to no good and was rather going to suffer severe setbacks in his mental faculties that would leave him permanently disabled and dependent. Flashbacks of such thoughts were quite frustrating and frightening to me, and I needed a way out.

Charles continued listening to me further, and then said, "Let me remind you of something". He got his phone and showed me certain scripture posters forwarded to him several months earlier. They were sent as highlights for a Bible Study discussion we had at our fellowship meetings in those days. Then he started asking me questions about what I remembered from the chapter study of 2 Corinthians 4. I honestly did not remember and thus could not say much then. But this is what the references we discussed say in the Living Bible.

2 Corinthians 4:7-18 reads as follows:

"But this precious treasure, this light and power that now shine within us, is held in a perishable container, that is in our weak bodies. Everyone can see that the glorious power within must be from God and is not our own. We are pressed on every side by troubles, but not crushed and broken. We are perplexed because we don't know why things happen as they do, but we don't give up and quit. We are hunted down, but God never abandons us. We are knocked down, but we get up again and keep going.

These bodies of ours are constantly facing death just us Jesus did, so it is clear to all that it is only the living Christ within who keeps us safe. Yes, we live under constant danger to our lives because we serve the Lord, but this gives us constant opportunities to show forth the power of Jesus Christ within our dying bodies. Because of our preaching we face death, but it has resulted in eternal life for you. We boldly say what we believe trusting God to care for us, just as the psalm writer did when he said "I believe and therefore I speak". We know that the same God who brought the Lord Jesus back from death will also bring us back to life again with Jesus and present us to Him along with you. These sufferings of ours are for your benefit. And the more of you who are won to Christ, the more there are to thank Him for His great kindness, and the more the Lord is glorified

That is why we never give up. Though our bodies are dying, our inner strength in the Lord is growing every day. These troubles and sufferings of ours are, after all, quite small and won't last very long. Yet this short time of distress will

This reminder and assurance was very revealing for me.
Charles urged me to keep reading and thinking about
these scriptures and remind God of them as often as my
thoughts and feelings were challenged. To him, it was
certain that I would face confrontation, intimidation
and temptation from the enemy as I continued to seek
God's intervention and breakthrough for my son. When
Charles was leaving me, I knew I had to calm down and
toughen up at the same time, whether through tears and
toil and trial, or through faith and aids and triumphs. I
assured myself that somehow it could be God's will for
my son to live with autism and, if so, he would eventually
make it. I eventually told myself to start training my mind
to look up and look beyond, to see God and see my son's
future, and also to build on my faith and hope in the
eventual outcome of his life.

Many years have gone by, but this word continues to
build a new kind of tranquility within my heart. From
my meditations on it, the Holy Spirit has led me to more
and more eternal truths. For instance I have learned that
to be tempted is not wrong, and one need not feel guilty
when tempted. Eve did not sin until she yielded (Genesis
3:6). David yielded to the temptation and sin of adultery
when he saw Bathsheba. Jesus was tempted, yet without

sin. I realize now that in Matthew 4:3 the real temptation was the suggestion to Jesus not to wait for God to provide for His dire need, but to act independently to provide for Himself. He very well overcame the devil here. Remember that Jesus indeed multiplied bread and fish to feed the five thousand people on the hillside. He also actually turned water into wine at the wedding in Cana. So Jesus had the power to do what the devil was demanding of Him very easily. But Jesus understood what the devil was doing by asking Him to turn stones into bread at the time when He, Jesus, was hungry and needed food (bread) as answer to His need. The test was to determine whose interest and ultimate will Jesus was going to pursue in that moment of need and for that matter in the ordinary causes of His life. Was Jesus going to seek His need at that time or was He going to obey God's Word, which was very well known to Him? Even if He could justify the need for food having fasted for forty days, was that time the moment when God wanted Him to seek food? Was it for Him to provide that food for and by Himself? Was the outcome of His having that need met at that moment what God had destined for Him within His mission on earth? These and many other questions arise when one reflects on the account of the temptation of Jesus Christ (Matthew 4).

It is often the case that when believers (as humans) are tempted to pray fervently for something, we then think that because it is a good request meant for our well-being and the glory of God's name, it must be granted as we wish. The temptation therefore is when we begin to focus on "I want what I want when I want it". The truth is that we sometimes ask for the right thing at the wrong time. Other times we ask for things without pausing to find out if indeed they are within the will of God for us. These are the actual reasons why we get frustrated with God's decision that we wait, for when we slip into such situations, Satan will come in with the fiercest of temptations. Satan hates us, just because God loves us so much so that we remind him of God when he seeks to focus on us. I have learnt from the Holy Spirit that the smart thing to do when we are faced with a seemingly impossible situation is to keep on praying.

A. W. Tozer has shared the view that *"a praying Christian is a constant threat to the stability of Satan's government. The Christian is a holy rebel loose in the world with access to the throne of God. Satan never knows from what direction the danger will come. Who knows when another Elijah will arise, or another Daniel? Or a Luther or a Booth? Who knows when an Edwards or a Finney may go in and liberate a whole town or countryside by preaching of the word and prayer. Such a danger is too great to tolerate, so Satan gets to the new convert as early as possible to prevent his becoming too formidable a foe".*

Because Satan dreads the potency and outcome of our prayers, he constantly deploys conditions such as frustration, fear, dejection and hopelessness against us to clutter our focus. I have learnt that we have a more compelling and powerful reason not to lose focus nor take our eyes off our hope and trust in the Lord in every situation. This reason is that we actually hold hands with a great host of unseen persons in unbroken chains of blessing. This blessed hope is what the Holy Spirit has been teaching me to make my focus and preoccupation always for some time now. He has given me insights into His word, for instance what **1 Peter 1:11-13** says. It reads as follows:

"Searching what or what manner of time the Spirit of Christ who was in them was indicating when He testified beforehand the sufferings of Christ and the glories that would follow. To them it was revealed that not to themselves, but to us they were ministering the things which now have been reported to you through those who have preached the gospel to you by the Holy Spirit sent from heaven, things which angels desire to look into. Therefore gird up the loins of your mind, be sober and rest your hope fully upon the grace that is to be brought to you at the revelation of Jesus Christ."

In living out my life with this hope I have come to appreciate how powerful a life of hope is. I personally know the truth as O.S. Marden puts it, that "there is no medicine like hope, no incentive so great, and no tonic as powerful as expectation of something tomorrow". This truth gives me so much strength and power to persevere through the tough times. **Shlomo Breznitz** has also said, that "Hope, if it is serious, if it is long term, leads to physiological changes that can improve the body's resistance. In our studies we have found two hormones, cortisol and prolactin, that are strongly affected by an attitude of hope. While we don't know the precise links, the evidence points to a strong relationship between such neurochemicals and the immune system. People with a strong faith, whether from religious beliefs or just good experience with trust, are the ones who stick it out in the worst circumstances".

If you are out there struggling to stay hopeful in life because of an impossible situation confronting you, I have a little to share with you. Hope is a powerful stimulant. I illustrate my belief in this truth as well by quoting from an essay titled "Hope Sprouts Eternal" published in the Time Magazine, January 28, 1985 edition. It reads:

"Without the power of hope, the world would be quite a different place. Christopher Columbus would probably have looked to the Western horizon and told his crew, 'There doesn't seem to be anything in sight, let's turn around and go home'. Military campaigns would have ended differently. George Washington, surveying his ragged forces at Valley Forge, would have surrendered. So would Winston Churchill in the early days of 1941. The march of industrial technology would have zigzagged. Thomas Edison after spending $40,000 to test umpteen hundred possible filaments for an electric light would have shrugged and said, 'I give up, nobody will ever figure this out'. Most of the heroes of literature would have been far less heroic".

Hope is God's gift to you to keep you healthy and positive and persevering. Even though hope often implies waiting for indefinite moments for the expectation of one's heart, it will eventually prove worthy of the wait. **George Matheson,** reflecting on 'why wait when you are hoping for something of eternal value' had this insightful comment to make, that *"we commonly associate patience with lying down. We think of it as the angel that guards the* *couch of the invalid. Yet there is patience that I believe to be harder, the patience that can run. To lie down in the time of grief, to be quiet under the stroke of adverse fortune implies a great strength. But I know of something that implies a strength greater still. It is the power to work under stress, to continue under hardship, to have anguish in your spirit and still perform daily tasks. This is a Christlike thing. The hardest thing is that most of us are called to exercise patience, not in the sick bed, but in the street."*

To further emphasize the importance of upholding hope in God with patience in suffering, Chris Tiegreen has said that "*those who rebel against their suffering, however, are still hoping in the here and now. Somewhere deep inside they had expected a better deal in this life and not yet invested their hopes in God's kingdom. They had an agenda for this life that didn't fit with His*".

Together with the foregoing quotations, I do share the thought that when despair and disillusionment cloud our focus we are like blind people. Everything becomes dark and gloomy. But remembering brings God's promises to the fore-front of our minds. God promises that all things will work together for good. Yes, God says He will work character, perseverance and hope in your life through these hard times. I also believe it takes courage to wait patiently and yet get out there and embrace life. But you can do it. Lean on God and courage will never be in short supply.

My reality of hope is that God gives a reason to hope every day, whether out of grief, or love, or repentance and the like, He brings peace, and hope that lasts forever.

SOLITUDE IN THE CHAOS

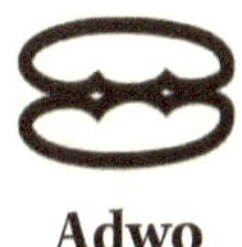

Adwo

"A man who cannot find tranquility within himself will search for it in vain elsewhere". Francois La Rochefoucauld.

This chapter is dedicated to honoring Bishop Joseph Garlington, an amazing preacher and excellent gospel musician. Bishop Garlington is Pastor of Covenant Church of Pittsburgh, PA, USA. I thank Bishop Garlington for helping me hear quite clearly again the voice of the Holy Spirit bringing me the instruction to sit a while with Him in silence, and in practising solitude, also benefit from His uplifting rest whenever the going gets tough in this life.

There was this day when my son Yooku suffered a meltdown at the airport of all places, in Accra. He was to travel to the United States with my Sheila (his mum) for a visit and certain medical reviews. We arrived at the airport and to an over-crowded departure lounge. After queuing for a long time, we got to the counter only to be informed that my son's passport was to expire in about three months, and so he needed to have it renewed before he could be allowed to travel with it across continents. The long waiting period had gotten my son already agitated and restless. As I was trying to get the flight authorities to consider a waiver of the regulation on medical grounds, we had to move to a couple of offices to consult the responsible immigration and aviation officers available. This process aggravated Yooku's agitation and before long he suffered a full blown meltdown. He started screaming and yelling. All manner of security officers came to us at the lounge. He attacked one man, kicking and biting him. I grabbed him and pinned him to the ground, but he kept screaming, and soon security officers came, intending to hand-cuff him. I pleaded with them not to and explained his condition to them. I was given a bind-belt to use to tie his hands to stop him from hitting us. I reached for a rope in his first aid bag and then tied his legs as well to stop him from kicking. I also inserted in his mouth an apparatus we used to stop him from biting himself and others.

By this time, he was on the ground in the lounge and we were surrounded by all manner of people. There was utter confusion. He was traumatized. He was drenched in sweat and looked awfully stressed. He continued screaming and stamping his bound feet on the floor. I managed to give him his oral pill meant for sedating him when that happened, and poured a bottle of water on his head and down his body. Even though Sheila and I understood what had happened to him, we felt anxious and helpless. We had to do everything possible to ensure that he did not injure himself or anybody else around us in that situation. In addition to the physical beating and manhandling both of us had suffered at his hand, we were both overwhelmed with shame and despair, knowing that we had suddenly become the talk of the crowd in the lounge. It was quite a depressing experience, and holding one's head high was very difficult at that moment.

I wish to say in direct connection and association with that incident, that sometimes the behaviour or reactions of the people in the immediate presence of the autistic person compounds their challenge. I believe people start talking, shouting, standing by to look on and at what is happening and so forth because of things like curiosity, anxiety, shock and confusion. But it is helpful when autistic persons suffer meltdowns, that they are isolated and or contained in open solitary spaces. That way they don't feel hemmed in or captured. For this reason, it is better for on-lookers to rather vacate the room, space or immediate environs where the autistic person is. The space and quiet this creates makes the healing and recovery from meltdowns faster. The feeling and sense of being left alone rather than captured helps them to calm down and accept themselves. Also, where the parent, guardian or care-giver with the autistic person is overwhelmed or appears physically overpowered, it is useful if a strong and firm person within their reach offers a bare hug to the autistic person, make gestures of acceptance and safety to him, and provide the needed support to help their recovery. Most autistic children experiencing meltdowns scream and cry out of pain and anxiety, and so a calming quiet presence, a welcoming shoulder, a friendly bare hug and sometimes a bottle of drinking water are all of valuable healing aid to them.

I have personally seen autistic children under stress meltdowns respond swiftly and positively to soft singing and humming of simple songs to them by the immediate neighbours around them. They are likely to sit up, look into their faces, smile or gesture to say thank you and them slowly pick themselves up again with normal behaviour. I humbly suggest that all of us in our varied social settings should try to help out where we can by doing such simple acts of sisterly care for them.

Back then that night, a Port Health official eventually came to us and helped us into a prepared side-room which had a sofa and some chairs. It was empty, and so we changed Yooku's clothes and tried to get him to calm down while lying on the sofa. I untied him and sat next to him, hoping that the first aid pill given him would help him gain a bit of calm and composure. It didn't really work, but after almost half an hour of screaming, stamping, hitting and so forth, he was naturally tired and began to slow down on his tantrums. Two other officers came to us with his passport and a formal notice that he and Sheila could travel on the next flight of the same airline two days later. We were then advised to use whatever expedited service that could be made available to us to have Yooku's passport renewal done within that two-day period. We waited there for some time, and when most of the check-in processes had ended and the counters had closed leaving the lounge almost vacated by the crowd, we left the airport and went back home, but to a long and confused night. We had to call and send messages to our host family in the United States about the flight challenges and the prospect of travel in two days.

The next morning Yooku had flu and was quite weak. We had to get him some medication, and we spent the day pursuing the business of getting him the renewed passport. Thankfully, we got a lot of assistance and were able to get all the processes done. I was able to pick up the new passport the following day at about two o'clock in the afternoon so travel was possible that evening. We consulted Yooku's doctor and got guidance on alternative medical preparation for him during the almost two-day travel period ahead of him and Sheila, and equipped his first aid bag with the necessaries. As a family, we had to pray and trust God for His tender mercies to see them through on the journey. Sheila was at peace with herself, knowing that God's grace was sufficient for their safety. We prayed and trusted God for a calm spirit and composure for Yooku throughout their journey and mission in the United States. They indeed had a safe flight and got home safely to their host family without any challenge. Our faithful God kept them in His peace and quiet, and all was well with them.

Two days after their trip was a Sunday, and I found myself in church for the forenoon service. I was still down in my spirit and felt wearied by the circumstances and events of the past few days. Uncertainty about my wife and son was very present on my mind. Sleep and rest could not come easily either. So I was in church that morning, hoping that God would meet my need for His rest and assurance that all would be well. Guess what! God had prepared for me. Bishop Joseph Garlington spoke the word of God directly and clearly to my spirit-man. He preached on the subject of God's elevation when we feel let down and out by life's circumstances, dwelling on Psalm 46.

As is very characteristic of Bishop Garlington, he took off with his sermon that morning, ministering powerfully in song. He sang the song, "You Raise Me Up" by Josh Groban in a wonderful way while Pastor Clarence, an associate of his, played the organ, seizing the presence in the auditorium for the Lord. He preached a practical message, pointing us to many ways and means by which God has lifted us from our fallen state. Then he admonished us passionately to believe that it is God's preoccupation to elevate us in this life, so that each Christian's testimony of His faithfulness would eternally honor Him. Midway through the sermon, Bishop Garlington just got the congregation upstanding with him and we sang the song twice together so purposefully before he asked us to take our seats. The amazing thing is that when we were singing together the line that says 'I am strong when I am on your shoulders', I heard the voice of the Holy Spirit say softly to me ***"You have my shoulder, so assure yourself of my word (Psalm 46) and keep going"***. My spirit and my face lightened up and I knew that was Him. I don't know how to describe it well, but the 'stillness' I felt was novel. What was more, the preacher finished singing and preaching, and then said, "*Whatever you heard while we sang, you better believe it, because you're already elevated*".

That was an amazing encounter, and I have lived with the pleasant memory of it for years now. The song says;

When I am down and, Oh my soul so weary
When troubles come and my heart burdened be
Then, I am still and wait here in the silence
Until You come and sit a while with me.
You raise me up, so I can stand on mountains
You raise me up, to walk on stormy seas
I am strong, when I am on your shoulders
You raise me up to more than I can be.

The next day I spent my lunch break from work at a beachfront location in Accra. Sitting all alone in that quiet place, I enjoyed the breeze and read over Psalm 46 several times to get it sinking into my mind. I was not intending to memorize it, but to get it into my thought-frame and belief. I wanted to obey the Holy Spirit's voice, but I also wanted to have to some degree the knowledge the sons of Korah who are reputed to have written this song of scripture had of God and His virtues, which they described so well. These are the words of the psalm.

"God is our refuge and strength, a very present help in trouble. Therefore we will not fear, even though the earth be removed, and though the mountains be carried into the midst of the sea. Though its waters roar and be troubled, though the mountains shake with its swelling. Selah

There is a river whose streams shall make glad the city of God, the holy place of the tabernacle of the Most High.

God is in the midst of her, she shall not be moved. God shall help her, just at the break of dawn. The nations raged, the kingdoms were moved, He uttered His voice, the earth melted. The Lord of hosts is with us, The God of Jacob is our refuge. Come, behold the works of the Lord, who has made desolation in the earth. He makes wars cease to the end of the earth. He breaks the bow and cuts the spear in two. He burns the chariot in the fire. Be still, and know that I am God. I will be exalted among the nations, I will be exalted in the earth. The Lord of hosts is with us. The God of Jacob is our refuge. Selah.

From that lunch appointment and my meditations thereafter, the following have been some of my lessons from Psalm 46 in particular and my perspectives on solitude in chaotic situations in general. First of all God is described as our refuge, strength, and very present help. From this I know that God is my refuge. I have thus assured myself that my refuge is in the Person of God. With that, I have also been telling myself often that whenever I have trouble coming my way, He is present to be my strength and help. So when I am down, weary, stressed, frustrated and or troubled in anyway, He is the Merciful One who bends down to listen to my cry for help and rescues me from those storms of life. For example, I see autism as an enemy. When any of the manifestations of autism makes life difficult for my son, I have to help him contain and compose himself so he does not end up hurting and harming himself. Sometimes he actually harms himself or hurts others, and that naturally leaves me stressed and confused, or tired and frustrated. In those moments, I run to God for refuge against this enemy, and His strength fights away from me despair and discouragement.

I am assured that the Holy Presence of the Most High God (described in verses 4 to 7) is always with me, and us, and is busy bringing to an end the elements of strife in our lives. The elements of the strife in the earth mentioned in the psalm include mountains, tsunamis, roaring waters, desolation, armors, chariots and fires. I can liken these to the anxieties, fears, depression, sorrows and despair that consistently strike us through the changing scenes of life. And Psalm 46 emphatically invites us to "be still and know" of our God in those contexts, that He is God, who will be exalted in the nations and in the earth (verse 10). The language of instruction used in this verse at the face level seems abstract, but I can assure you it is very practical if you are indeed approaching it with true obedience. To '**be still**' means to be **quiet and stable** in the midst of the chaos and confusion. To 'know' here means to understand and accept that something (for example an event or statement) is factual and true. From my personal and practical obedience of this instruction, I am totally assured that God is never withdrawn from me when I am troubled and tempted to give up. He always presents Himself to me as exalted above my trouble and then provides me with His help and strength to prevail and overcome. He is always present to comfort and raise me up from any situation that makes me feel left below and under the current.

Learning more about this discipline, I have come across Henri Nouwen's thought about practicing solitude. He says in his published work *Making All Things New* (1981), *"we are usually surrounded by so much inner and outer noise that it is hard to truly hear our God when He is speaking to us. We have often become deaf. Thus our lives become absurd, in which word we find the Latin word "surdus", meaning deaf. A spiritual discipline is necessary in order to move slowly from an absurd to an obedient life, from a life filled with noisy worries to a life in which there is some free inner space"*

This has proved very useful and beneficial to me. Every now and again, the Holy Spirit helps me to consciously close my ears and mind to the noisy clutter and distractions that autism regularly brings into the lives of families and individuals. The better reality is also that He, the Holy Spirit, speaks to me in the quiet of my heart when I open up to hear from Him, especially soon after all the disturbing behaviors of my son stop.

Anne & Ray Ortlund have explained in their book *Staying Power* (1986) that *"when you've gotten rid of your outer distractions, you may become very aware of your inner distractions, the anxieties, the bad memories, the anger and the chaos of your heart. Maybe for a few weeks your solitude will not only seem a waste, but even painful"*.

Personally, I am assured that it pays to be deliberately quiet. When you refuse to feed or pay attention to the outer and inner distractions, they will gradually withdraw from you. When you remain quiet, the Holy Spirit brings in His inner peace, and you'll become aware of God and eternity. You realize that your personality can be stripped-down, quieted and unburdened. As mentioned earlier on in this book, the Lord Jesus' instruction to the disciples in Mark 6:31, thus "come with me by yourselves to a quiet place and get some rest" is so simple and practical that every christian should be able to practise it in obedience to Him. I explain below what exactly I mean by practising in obedience to Jesus Christ this little instruction.

We must all as believers learn to withdraw from our routines and create a little quietude in our lives from time to time to be able to listen in to the voice of God. In carrying out our tiring daily duties, we must sometimes decisively take a short break and seek rest in the Presence of the Lord. This is best done in quiet places. In the quiet places, Jesus does not only give us rest, but He also teaches us how to depend on Him more fully. He teaches us how to serve Him more effectively, and how to serve Him more implicitly. The quiet places are places of growth, where we deepen our fellowship with Him, and instead of a temporary rest, we have a relationship that will continue to sustain us when the pressures of life are up against us. The things we learn in the calm with the Holy Spirit are the things that will help us survive in the storms ahead.

Anne & Ray Ortlund say further that *"the more we train ourselves to spend time with God and Him alone, the more we discover that God is with us at all times and in all places.*

Once the solitude of time and space has become a solitude of the heart, we will never have to leave that solitude. We will be able to live the spiritual life in any place and any time. Thus the discipline of solitude enables us to live active lives in the world, while remaining always in the presence of the living God".

I dare say, that there is within us and beyond the realm of our conscious knowledge, a divine life under His loving care. There is a controlling presence the Holy Spirit brings into one's life which works in stillness. It is never wearied nor exhausted, but controls our whole being, and transforms us into the image of God. This is the benefit of our deliberate practice of solitude in His presence, and I can testify that this has been of immense help to me and my family in our experiences of managing lives challenged by autism. That is why I agree completely with what Linda Dillow also says about practicing solitude in her reflections on Psalm 46. She says that *"you need a place to hide when life overwhelms you, and scripture promises that God Almighty will be your refuge and fortress. When your personal world seems out of control, the glorious promises of Psalm 46 are just what you need"*.

KENYAN BOY'S DILEMMA

Nyame Nwu Na M'ewu

*Rarely do we view the difficult circumstances of life as statements of Jesus' love for us. We more likely interpret them as interruptions in our walk with God. In our best moments, we may interpret these interruptions as tools God will use to stretch our faith; in our worst moments, we may even see them as His disfavor. But we still tend to view them as distractions from the course He would have us pursue. **Chris Tiegreen**.*

I pay my tribute for this chapter to a Kenyan boy whose full name I do not know. Let me conveniently identify him as Shadrack, even though his first name was given in my source story. I have not met him, but I very much wish to meet him someday in life. I do know, however, that this boy is autistic, and lived alone with his mother Lucy in a quiet neighborhood in Kenya's countryside. Why pay tribute to him is a question I will answer along the way in the chapter.

20th June 2019 will continue to be a memorable day in my life for all the unusual reasons. It is recorded in my living memory as one very dark day because of what happened to me after learning of this Kenyan boy's experience. I experienced massive sorrow and fear at the same time, and I could not keep my head or my spirit up. That night was surely one of the longest I have known all my life, filled with grief and helplessness. I could neither wish away the night nor hope for the morning, it was all gloom and despair in my heart and around me. I could not even pray.

On this day I saw and read a post on a social media platform I share in. It was a short story about someone I call Shadrack, a Kenyan boy known to be autistic. The report said he lived alone with his mother in a quiet neighborhood, and did not attend school, probably because there was no special school in his area with a curriculum and training system which could be suitable for him. Nothing was said about his father or siblings. But he was known to join his mother in the market and community business enclave where she worked. He was said to be about nine years old. He had no verbal speech, no regular friends, and was said to manifest autistic behaviors such as screaming, flapping his hands, chewing plastics, frequent unprovoked laughing, kicking and biting.

Shadrack was in the news, I mean social media reportage that day because he had come out of his home with loud screams and unusual noise, onto the street and all he was attempting to do was to drag anybody he could see out there into the house where he lived. The neighbors had not seen his mother for three days, even though he was always in the company of his mother. The report said he was ignored by several people he tried to drag along with him, and he kept on running in and out of the house. He went and brought out some of his mother's clothes and threw them onto the street amid loud cries. Eventually, two women went to him, and he characteristically pointed to the house, dragging them in with him. They went in to discover that his mother had died, probably two or three days earlier, and he was all morning just trying to draw someone's attention to this and seek help. How sad. The report said the women aroused public attention and helped to bring in the appropriate public authorities, family and professional neighbors to take care of the body and truncate the boy's traumatic situation.

This stunning story traumatized me and threw me into a state of grief. Being a parent of a boy with autism, I found myself asking many questions. Maybe these were legitimate, maybe unnecessary, but as they say 'the more I ask the less I know'. I ended up imagining what was to happen to that boy Shadrack. Knowing from my experiences with my own son how demanding and interruptive an autistic child can be, I was wondering how that boy was going to find acceptance, tolerance and comfort from a new set of family and care-giving neighbours, be they already known or unknown to him. Among my many questions were?

1. How long had the mother been dead?
2. Did Shadrack know or realize she was dead?
3. What had he tried to do to help her survive her last moments?

4. Did she tell him anything at all before she died?

5. What did she tell him then?

6. What did he understand whatever he may have been told to mean?

7. What did he think was going to happen to him?

8. Was there any real family out there for him?

9. How was he going to live without his mother?

10. How was his obvious trauma going to be treated?

11. Did he really understand what had happened?

12. Could he trust whoever (ie social workers, nurses, foster parents etc) were to help him in his new life?

13. Would Shadrack have a stable mind and grow up into a sane adult?

My list could be much longer, but somehow I accepted the fact that legitimate or not my questions were not going to be answered in any practical way. I gave up questioning, but I could not stop thinking and agonizing about Shadrack. I thought about devoting myself to pray continually for that boy, but I did not even know what to pray for. I was truly overcome by anxiety and grief at every thought of this most troubled boy. I was also burdened because I could easily assume, from my experiences with my own son, that Shadrack could not meaningfully pray for himself. Thankfully, something Madame Guyon (a German poet who is reputed to have written many inspiring poems during her time in prison detention) had published came to mind and provided me with the right inspiration. Madame Guyon's statement reads as follows;

"When one loves what God is doing in one's life, one cannot hate the instrument through which it comes. Paul wrote many of his epistles in prison cells, John wrote the Book of Revelation while in exile, John Bunyan penned Pilgrim's Progress in the Bedford jail, Martin Luther translated the German Bible as a prisoner in Warburg Castle. Similarly, walking through seasons of pain has been the schoolroom where I have gone deeper in knowing the Holy One as the Blessed Controller of all things. Intimacy with my Bridegroom has blossomed in the prison of pain".

Thinking about this brought my prayer focus onto God's protection and provision for Shadrack as he goes through his own season of overwhelming pain and loneliness as a child, so that whatever the purposes of his loss and his very life would not be lost to him or abandoned. I welcomed the thought that God could reveal through the circumstances of his loss, His love for him as well as His unique assignment for him in this life, such that he would be fully committed to His use. That gave me a compelling reason and focus for prayer for him. In a few days I got an idea to add Shadrack to a list of persons I used to pray for in those days on Sunday mornings before going to church. These were old and sick persons who I knew could not get about easily and were left at home most of the time. I prayed for healing and protection from God for them. For the most part, I dwelt on Psalm 143 for guidance in prayer for them, and that gave me great hope and comfort in the Lord for Shadrack as well. This is what Psalm 143 says;

"Hear my prayer, O Lord. Listen to my plea. Answer me because You are faithful and righteous. Don't put your servant on trial, for no one is innocent before you. My enemy has chased me. He has knocked me to the ground and forces me to live in darkness like those in the grave. I am losing all hope; I am paralyzed with fear. I remember the days of old. I ponder all your great works and think about what you have done. I lift my hands to you in prayer. I thirst for you as parched land thirsts for rain. Come quickly, Lord, and answer me, for my depression deepens. Don't turn away from me, or I will die. Let me hear of your unfailing love each morning, for I am trusting you. Show me where to walk, for I give myself to you. Rescue me from my enemies, Lord; I run to you to hide me. Teach me to do your will, for you are my God. May your gracious Spirit lead me forward on a firm footing. For the glory of your name, O Lord, preserve my life. Because of your faithfulness, bring me out of this distress. In your unfailing love, silence all my enemies and destroy all my foes, for I am your servant".

For weeks, I remotely aligned Shadrack's name with verse three of this psalm and made it his heartbeat in prayer to God. I was certain that he had a life of darkness ahead of him, and so I interceded for him that God would draw him out of that darkness and bring him into His light that loves and leads. I was very comforted to see verse eight of this psalm as well. I had so much hope that for the fact that these two verses are together in one psalm, God must have dealt with this problem with several humans, and thus would be doing it again whilst I prayed. I had no way of knowing or deliberately checking on this boy to find out how he was doing and how things were turning out for him. But I was so burdened for him, and interceding for him came very easily to me. I remember one day I prayed and asked God for a picture of how He was holding that boy to Himself and guaranteeing his safety. This is because I know how boys with autism can so often put themselves in harm's way. In fact from my experience, one has to be looking out for them all the time to ensure that even in their own rooms and known environments they are not harming themselves with familiar objects, or through behaviors like biting, head-butting and kicking stuff around them. I have not seen that virtual picture as yet, but interestingly after about a year from that time, I have read and visualized God's love, provision and protection for people like Shadrack in scriptures such as the following.

*"You are my hiding place; You shall preserve me from trouble. You shall surround me with songs of deliverance. I will instruct you and teach you the way you should go; I will guide with My eye." (**Psalm 32:7-8**)*

*"He will feed his flock like a shepherd. He will gather the lambs with His arm, And carry them in His bosom, And gently lead those who are with young." (**Isaiah 40:11**)*

*"For in the time of trouble He shall hide me in His pavilion; In the secret place of His tabernacle He shall hide me; He shall set me high upon a rock" (**Psalm 27:5**)*

"Look at the birds of the air, for they neither sow nor reap

*nor gather into barns; yet your heavenly Father feeds them. Are you not of more value than they?" (**Matt. 6:26**)*

From these scriptures and more, I have gained more faith, confidence and comfort. I believe that Shadrack is not lost or abandoned to the dangers of living a homeless life without any guidance. I believe God has provided for him the needs of his life to guarantee his safety physically, mentally and spiritually. I have some peace within when I think about him or pray for him these days. I remember that exactly a year after I learnt about this boy and got upon myself this burden of praying for him, I read from **Isaiah 26:12(a),** which reads as follows; *"Lord, you have established peace for us".* This verse made more meaning to me when I also read a commentary on it by the legendary Alexander Maclaren, who wrote thus *"there is peace that comes from submission, tranquility of spirit, which is the crown and reward of obedience; repose which is the very smile upon the face of faith, and all these things are given unto us along with the grace and mercy of our God. And the man that possesses this is at peace with God and at peace with himself, so he may bear in his heart that singular blessing of a perfect tranquility and quiet amidst the distractions of duty, of sorrows, of losses and of cares".* The combined effect and benefit of knowing this truth from the scripture and understanding from faithful men has been that I have gained some peace in my thoughts about Shadrack, which peace has remained with me to date.

I am all the more encouraged about Shadrack and his well-being when I ponder the fact that the age-old famous hymn by Charles Wesley, "Gentle Jesus meek and mild" was inspired by the story of a little boy who fled his home and went hiding from a father who wanted him to go stealing for a living at the tender age of ten. He had learnt from his Sunday school teacher that stealing was a sin against the law of God and would not ever engage in it. This lad had total confidence in the Lord Jesus to take care of him and provide for him, so he sought to hide in Him alone. He lived a solitary life in an abandoned old building and unfortunately died a poor little boy, but he still has that hymn as part of his inspired legacy for the world today. Please brood over the lyrics of this hymn below and let it sink into your spirit for your own growth and fellowship with the Holy Spirit. Personally, I have immense inner peace now about Shadrack. I believe the good Lord is taking great care of him, providing for him and protecting him from every possible danger this world presents to him. I have that peace because the Faithful One has assured me that He holds His own, and will never leave nor forsake them. I am very grateful to the Holy Spirit for Shadrack, and the peace He has given me for his sake. My reflection on this story reveals to me that the life of faith requires us to lean on an invisible source of strength and wisdom. As we trust God, we find that very real and visible storms of life come up against our faith in Him, and yet He remains invisible. At some point in your walk of faith, you must learn to detach yourself from the things that concern you, and cast them wholly on God, believing that His gracious care is enough to handle them all.

1 .Gentle Jesus, meek and mild
Look upon a little child
Pity my simplicity
Suffer me to come to Thee

2. Fain I would to Thee be brought
Dearest God forbid it not
Give me, dearest God a place
In the kingdom of Thy grace

3. Put Thy hands upon my head
Let me in Thine arms be stayed
Let me lean upon Thy breast
Lull me, lull me Lord to rest

4. Hold me fast in Thy embrace
Let me see Thy smiling face
Give me Lord Thy blessing give
Pray for me, and I shall live.

5. I shall live the simple life
Free from sin's uneasy strife
Sweetly ignorant of ill
Innocent and happy still

6. O that I may never know
What the wicked people do
Sin is contrary to Thee
Sin is the forbidden tree

7. *Keep me from the great offense*
Guard my helpless innocence
Hide me from all evil hide
Self, and stubbornness and pride

8. *Lamb of God I look to You*
Thou shalt my Example be
Thou art gentle, meek and mild
Thou wast once a little child

9. *Fain I would be as Thou art*
Give me thine obedient heart
Thou art pitiful and kind
Let me have Thy loving mind.

10. *Meek and lowly may I be*
Thou art all humility
Let me to my betters bow
Subject to Thy parents Thou

11. *Let me above all fulfill*
God my heavenly Father's will
Never His good Spirit grieve
Only to His glory live

12. *Thou didst live to God alone*
Thou didst never seek Thine own
Thou Thyself didst never please
God was all Thy happiness

13. Loving Jesus, gentle Lamb
In Thy gracious hands I am
Make me Savior, what Thou art
Live Thyself within my heart

14. I shall then show forth Thy praise
Serve Thee all my happy days
Then the world shall always see
Christ, the holy Child, in me.

WAILING ON THE MOTORWAY

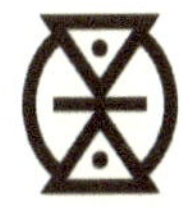

Mmere Dane

God tries our faith so that we may try His faithfulness, and He always succeeds in proving Himself as Lord of our situation. Anonymous.

When my son entered the adolescent stage, he became violent. It was almost a daily occurrence for him to attack somebody at home, at school, in church, at the hospital or out somewhere else. He often made someone his target for the day and would repeatedly hit that person, sometimes bite when that person was not watching, and also kick people from behind. We sought medical attention and explanations for this new development. We were advised on certain dietary changes and given medicines to help control his hormonal influxes, but the behaviors continued. Within a particular term of the school year in 2015, he attacked four of the care-givers in his school and physically assaulted them. His assaults left three of them with very bad bite-wounds that required tetanus injections. The Centre sought to manage this situation by changing his care-givers randomly each week, so that the possible fixation on any particular person to make his target could be defeated. Sadly this intervention and several other management strategies did not work. This was very worrisome and troubling for all of us as a family.

One morning Yooku attacked me while we were riding to his school. I pulled off the road, tied his hands and gave him a dose of his sedative medicine to help calm him down. We went on to his school, and when I removed the bandage-tie to free his hands, all hell broke loose. He smashed louvre blades, broke chairs and terrorized me together with four of the young men serving as care-givers at the Centre. This trauma was so intense, so we had to tie him up again, arms and legs, and I took him to see one of the doctors we consult on his autistic condition/issues. He was treated and discharged. I took him back home. At the hospital, while he was being stabilized in the ward, I had a discussion with the doctor. I got to understand a number of things which were likely to happen to my son during his adolescent years because of his special condition and also as a result of some of the medicines he was taking. I proceed below to share a few of them which were explained to me by the doctor and others I consulted, as well as what I learnt from my personal research on the subject with you.

I was told my son was experiencing what is called intermittent explosive disorder (IED). It is another mental health diagnosis, a collection of violent, out of control and unpredictable behaviors. It is also described as impulsive-control disorder. It is the inability to resist aggressive impulses to cause destruction and harm to others by children with developmental disabilities and other persons with conduct concerns.

I understood and appreciated the fact that some people with autism will have seizures. Approximately one in four persons will have seizures during puberty. Though the reason for this is not actually known, it is believed it may be due to hormonal changes in the body, or the side effects of medications. The causes include high fever, high and low sugar, alcohol and drug withdrawal. Anything that interrupts the normal connections between nerve cells in the brain can also cause a seizure. The first signs of seizures in persons with autism include long staring, stiffening of the body, loss of consciousness, sudden falling, breathing problems, fear and euphoria.

Because of a generalized sensitivity in many individuals with autism, their senses are impacted to a far greater extent than the average person's. Children who struggle to assimilate in this way may also have the diagnosis of integration disorder. I learnt later from a publication on Mental Health by William Stillman, that "genetics aside, anyone who has trouble communicating, sustaining social connections, and expressing pain or sensory sensitivities and who doesn't consistently have his or her intellect presumed would become depressed. If you have ever experienced a prolonged and debilitating condition, such as speech or mobility loss, you may be able to better empathize with such feelings of hopelessness and low self-esteem. A child is likely to first begin showing signs of depression on the precipice of adolescence."

After knowing about all these possibilities and the recent experiences of violence then, we had to learn new strategies to keep Yooku safe and improve our alertness so we could monitor his mood swings better for attention. As a family we had to pray a lot for him, and also called on some good relatives to continue praying with us for the grace, wisdom and strength to cope. We kept praying for Yooku to be saved from possible seizures and any sustained stress disorders. This went on for some time, but the attack episodes persisted, and smashing of doors, plates and various toys and play objects continued unabated. We went to have a head region and brain scan done for him, and thankfully the result showed he was free from likely seizures.

It turned out however that the worse was yet to come. For some reason, Yooku developed a fixation for grabbing and biting ladies' arms. He attacked his mother so often that she had to resort to wearing arm bands and tubes to protect herself when at home with him. He would so unexpectedly grab her hand and bite her that she could not take chances. On some occasions he would kick his junior brother very hard. There were days both of them had to stay within their rooms with doors locked for some time to be safe from his sudden attacks. I personally had to physically restrain him many times to subdue and bind him in order to apply his medication and calm him down.

During this phase, I had occasions to give up everything and stay at home alone with him for days just to attempt a break in his fixation on some of the ladies at his school for his targeted attacks. The intermittent nature of these meltdowns and violent attacks made it quite difficult for us as parents and the managers of the school to accurately manage him. We actually adopted several methods, some of which eventually worked out for him. One smart method which proved effective for him was the 'buddy system'. He was assigned as his buddy one very strong (well built) young man called Kwame who had just come in for his youth (national) service. The two of them became good friends and he was his only instructor for one whole term. In those days, I had to hand Yooku over to Kwame each morning and he spent his day with Kwame alone. Kwame took him through his numeracy, literacy, art and craft lessons and play sessions every day, and he did quite a good job at keeping him away from everybody else. They spent most of the days outside the classrooms and under a tree in the compound, and this worked quite well for Yooku. Gradually, whatever was getting his eyes fixed on the ladies as target objects for hitting and biting stopped. He did not stop and has not totally stopped hitting and biting, but what has changed significantly is that ladies are no more his prime target, and the frequency of the attacks has declined considerably.

However, certain other events from the phase described above put me in a very dangerous situation. Two Peace Corps volunteer workers happened to have been at Yooku's school in a particular week as part of their international exchange programme. He attacked both of them and left them with blood-stained arms from his bites. It was painful for me when I had to meet with them to apologise for my son's unfortunate actions. Thankfully, one of them was so gracious, and even consoled me, assuring me that they knew that getting bitten or attacked by an autistic child was possible. These volunteers knew this from previous experiences while handling autistic children back home in their country, so they were not traumatized. I felt really sorry and dismayed by all these developments in my son's life.

The following week another young lady research student, Selassie, suffered Yooku's attack during lunch break at the school. She was an autism care professional pursuing further studies. She waited for me and had a long conversation with me when I went to pick up my son at close of day. It was this lady who explained to me for the first time what could be the scientific reason for Yooku's targeting of ladies for the attacks and biting. She said one of the confirmed findings of studies into the intermittent explosive disorder (IED) manifestations among teenage boys with autism was that they were experiencing sexual urges and engaging in them by acting out their biting for relief. She also told me that one of the end-stage signs of the IED would be that Yooku might engage in repeated roars, most likely in the evenings before he falls asleep, and would stop by himself after some time.

In fact I was grief stricken at this, and felt very helpless. I wished there was just anything I could possibly do to help my son and save him from all those embarrassing difficulties he was going through. Selassie graciously shared with me some strategies to help minimize the severity of the situation and provide him some respite.

The following were some of the strategies she shared with me:

a) Remain calm when he throws tantrums, and ensure that he does not read signs of despair, and even where he gets upset, do not flare up in reaction to him

b) Speak directly to him in a low and unemotional tone of voice

c) Use visual signs and words of comfort to assure him of his safety

d) Gently guide him out of the place by touches like stroking, hugging and walking hand in hand with him.

e) Engage him in deep breathing to help him de-escalate.

With all these things happening in our lives, we started a long fast to call on our God for help. The thoughts and feelings were overwhelming for us, and we could only think of help from the Lord. Instead of doing what **I Peter 5:7** says, "Cast all your anxiety on Him because He cares for you", I was carrying a heavy burden of anxiety. I was afraid that Yooku could just suffer a seizure anytime one of those days. I was fretful that maybe he would attack somebody again who might not be as gracious and forgiving as the volunteers had been, and that could lead to ramifications we were not ready for. I sometimes felt the school might just ask me to withdraw him, and I dreaded what that would leave me with, because he had already been thrown out of one regular school and another school where he was on an inclusive programme for special needs children. I was also sufficiently troubled that he had made my home less safe for both my wife and my younger son.

I was on the motorway to Tema, Ghana's industrial city, one day during this period. While praying as I drove I was overtaken by grief and started wailing and weeping to the Lord. Quite unaware I was going through an emotional breakdown, I lost control of the car. In a split moment I heard several car-horns blurring around me. That alerted me and helped me get composed again. Thankfully, I was able to get off the road and park safely on the shoulder. All alone out there, I cried out my heart to my God, poured my fears and sorrows about my son's condition onto Him and asked Him to take the burden away. I don't really know how I got my work done in Tema that day, but the Lord saw me through and took me back home. My devotion the next day brought me the blessing of reading this scripture.

"Rejoice in the Lord always. Again I will say, rejoice.
Let your gentleness be known to all men. The Lord is at hand.

Be anxious for nothing, but in everything by prayer and supplication, with thanksgiving, let your requests be made known to God;

And the peace of God, which surpasses all understanding, will guard your hearts and minds through Christ Jesus." (**Philippians 4:4-7)**

I took this word with me for my meditation throughout the period of fasting, and I received considerable insight from the Holy Spirit. Let me share and explain a few of them to you now. The Lord Jesus promised us His peace. He packaged it like this in **John 14:27**, *"Peace I leave with you, My peace I give to you, not as the world gives do I give to you. Let not your heart be troubled, neither let it be afraid"*. This same peace is what the Apostle Paul wrote about to the Philippians and indeed all believers in Philippians 4:6-7, before inviting us to meditate on the eight eternal virtues (verse 8). One beautiful insight the Holy Spirit gave me from here is that to have this peace which is not from this world, we must decisively put off anxiety, as one puts off his shirt. One must remove anxiety from one's body, soul and spirit and place it somewhere else. It must be a deliberate conscious decision which a believer continuously practices as a habit.

A second thing we must strategically practice is prayer with thanksgiving. The strategy is that we must pray thanking God for definite needs He has provided. These definite needs provided are what we see listed in the Lord's Prayer. **Matthew 6:9-13** clearly shows the list has two parts; namely God's needs and man's need.

God's needs in our prayer of thanksgiving come first, and they are to hallow and praise to His name, the coming of His kingdom, and the doing of His will on earth as it is in heaven. Man's needs come second, and they are His giving us our daily bread, His forgiveness of our sins/ debts, His leading us away from temptation, and His deliverance from evil and satan's power.

The explanation is that the Holy Spirit prompts us to pray with thanksgiving but not only when we are well and good and feeling blessed with all the physical and spiritual goodies we love. We must also equally and daily be filled with gratitude and pray thanking God, especially when we have crisis situations in our lives. This meets the needs of God, because we reflect that we remember the faithful supplies of His goodness in the past, we show that we are submitted to His sovereignty in the present, and also say that we can trust Him as sufficient for our future. The scriptures in **I Thessalonians 5:15-18** and **Jeremiah 32:16-44** confirm this.

Thirdly, we must dwell on God's promise of His peace in our lives in order to be able to enjoy it. We must do this by maintaining an intimate, continuous and deepening relationship with God for His peace. We must seek to please Him in our thoughts, with our words and our deeds.

I have learnt through these circumstances and from the leading of the Holy Spirit that instead of being anxious, the Lord expects us to draw near to Him as the God of our peace, focus on His grace in the Lord Jesus Christ, pour out our hearts' requests in prayer, and He will respond by guarding our hearts and minds through Christ Jesus. This is His definite standard of the attitude we must have all the time regardless of the circumstances, and the surest way we can practice that is to "Rejoice Always".

FAITH IN THE FUTURE.

Nsoromma

I dedicate this chapter to Nick Vujicic. This Australian young man was born with very serious deformities, and yet exudes so many abilities and capabilities that he is very deserving of every accolade an inspirational motivational speaker anywhere in the world can be given. I pay my tribute to him here because he is the one single individual who has moved me from having hope for the future to having faith in the future of my son, and for that matter all children with autism. In his book titled **Life Without Limits** (2010) Nick Vujicic makes the emphatic statement, while reflecting on a missed opportunity to go on a mission to India, thus; *"I believe God has a plan we cannot see. That is why it is so important to have faith in the future and to keep working toward your goals even when the odds seem stacked against you."*

Nick is a young man born without limbs. In his publications and motivational speeches around the world, he has so forcefully told the broken hearted, disabled and deformed persons across the world that *"there is great power in believing in your destiny"*. I have chosen to discuss this and other statements by Nick at this point because I found his perspective on the trio of

disability, destiny and **purpose** most insightful and more conclusive than anything else I have personally ever read on the subject. I will tell you what I mean and why I think this way in a moment. The description "born with it or born like that" is often used for persons/children with autism. As a parent, I can say that no matter how long and how hard one tries to come to terms with that reality, it is difficult to accept it without any denial or a lingering thought that perhaps one's sins or inactions may be responsible for the disability. It is common for parents of autistic children to slip into self-pity, blaming one's self or others or even God for their child's predicament. It is almost as though you can never escape from being questioned either directly or inadvertently about how your child was born with autism, and society very often deems it convenient to hold parents responsible for such.

Generally speaking, it is easy to ignore this notion and treatment, or get used to it as a usual attitude. This is because it is in the nature of man to ask why. Whenever we see tragedy in our world we tend to ask why. When we encounter hardship in our lives, or suffer loss, we ask why. We want to know the reason for it all, and the unifying purpose behind this strange, needy world. What we often fail to realize is that the universe exists to display the unique and singular splendor of God, as the scripture says in Revelation 4:11. But the truthful reality is that even though we can't help but think that this universe is about us as humans, it is not. That is why when life is hard on us, it doesn't make sense.

From my personal experience in the Ghanaian society, I dare to say that quite a few people have made up their minds and believe that having an autistic child is a curse. Others insist parents must have done something untoward to deserve their child. This is something that is intriguing, because I chose and engaged one or two of such people. I found out they were very uninformed scientifically about autism and other neuro-challenging conditions. I must say though that I have largely ignored the comments and opinions of people who have directly or indirectly spoken to me about the source, cause and supposed reasons for why one in this society would have a child with autism. But as I have said earlier, I find the attitude and perspective of Nick Vujicic inspirational and thus worth discussing. In fact I strongly recommend Nick's publications and television programmes to others. Beginning with Jesus' encounter with and healing of the man born blind in John's Gospel chapter 9, Nick tells his story and makes known his outlook beyond his disability in a way that is profound. First, let us take a look at the story in John's gospel chapter 9. It reads as follows:

"Now as Jesus passed by, He saw a man who was blind from birth. And His disciples asked Him saying, Rabbi, who sinned, this man or his parents, that he was born blind?"

*Jesus answered: Neither this man nor his parents sinned, but that the works of God should be revealed in him. I must work the works of Him who sent Me while it is day, the night is coming when no one can work. As long as I am in the world, I am the light of the world." **John 9:1-5.***

Nick tells in his published speeches how this portion of the gospel impacted his life, because he had been asking himself the same question that the disciples of Jesus put to Him. He says that at age fifteen he was very well aware of his different personality and deformities or disability, and how that made him reliant on others. But he also realized from Jesus' answer to His disciples that he was not a burden, a curse, a misfortune or a punishment to anybody. He saw himself as having many possibilities in God's hands. He saw from Jesus' answer that he was not even deficient in any way, but a custom-made person for God's works to be made manifest in him and in his generation. What I find most profound is what Nick says about God's purpose for him. He says in his book **Life Without Limits** that "*when I read that Bible verse at age fifteen, a <u>wave of peace</u> swept over me as I'd never known before. I'd been questioning why I was born without limbs, but now I realized that the answer was unknowable to anyone but God. I simply had to accept that and believe in the possibilities that He would present for me*"

Because of Nick's statement, I now believe that there are things God has probably purposed for no one to know about, just as in the case of the blind man in John's gospel. That means the questions and accusations, suspicions and blame from others are all unimportant and unfounded. What is important and worth seeking answers for is what Jesus has to say about His works and his purpose that is to be revealed in a disabled and or challenged person who has different abilities and circumstances.

Furthermore, Nick says about the scripture (John 9:1-5) that "*those words gave me a **sense of joy** and a feeling of strength. For the first time I realized that the fact that I* *couldn't understand why I have no limbs didn't mean that my Creator had abandoned me. The blind man was healed to serve His purpose. I wasn't healed, but my purpose in His grand purpose would be revealed in time. You must understand that sometimes in life you won't get the answers you seek right away. You have to walk by faith. I had to learn to trust in the possibilities for my life. If I can have that trust, you can too. The hard times and the discouragements are not fun. You don't have to pretend to enjoy them. But believe in the possibilities for better days ahead, for a fulfilling and purposeful life."* _

As I have said earlier Nick has said very emphatically in various words that there is an answer that cannot be made known to us about everyone, and for that matter one must have faith in the future. This, in my view, must be over and above the hope we often live by, because it is not founded or determinable from within us and our life's circumstances. It has to be derived from the purpose of Jesus Christ as the Creator, and the works of God which He seeks to reveal in each individual He has placed here on earth.

I must confess that sometimes I still think about and wonder what will become of my son, and by extension the children with autism I see living in my country. This is because the current public policy for the education and eventual assimilation of children with autism into the larger society is very scanty and quite redundant. With the very dynamic nature of the behaviors of children with autism, and lack of the consistent investment required for providing the needed personnel and range of training facilities for their purposes, it is quite unsettling to envision a future for them. But I can say that after I was alerted to faith in the future by Nick, the destiny of these children is not as blurred to me anymore. What they are made for and would become is firmly in God's hands, well set within His grand plan.

The subject of the future is one that many thinkers and men of faith have made plain for humanity; yet one has to be selective all the time to be right about it. What I have found very helpful in this regard is that one has a choice to be consistently positive and focused on the possibilities, and that way the negativities that any disability presents get faded out. I have been motivated by reading more about the subject, and I share a few of the great ideas I have gained. The venerable Oswald Chambers in his publication **"My Utmost For His Highest"** advises that fretting always ends in sin. He said *"We imagine that a little anxiety and worry are an indication of how really wise we are; it is much more an indication of how really wicked we are. Fretting comes from a determination to get our own way. Our Lord never worried and He was never anxious, because He was not out to realize His own ideas. He was out to realize God's ideas"*. Chambers' opinion is further stated thus, *"If you can see God using some lives, but into your life an obstacle has come and you do not seem to be of any use, keep paying attention to the Source, and God will either take you round it or remove it. Never get your eyes on the obstacle or on the difficulty"*.

According to President Abraham Lincoln, *"The best thing about the future is that it comes only one day at a time. God gives us the vision, then He takes us down to the valley to batter us into the shape of the vision, and it is in the valley that so many of us faint and give way. Every vision will be made real if we will have patience. God has to take us into the valley, and put us through fires and floods until we get to the place where He can trust us with the veritable reality."*

The Holy Spirit requires us to deal with issues emanating from this situation of blame from fellow humans for what God has done to reveal Himself in another person's life. I was awakened one night with a strong urge to read and study **Jeremiah 29**, so I did so. It was then that the Holy Spirit opened the eyes of my understanding to that ultimate purpose which He intends to implement with every challenged life that truly believes in Him in spite of the challenge. This is how I would like to state it.

First of all, I learnt from reading and studying Jeremiah 29 that God dealt with the nation and whole generation of Israel by maintaining His promise to them, but He never revealed and fulfilled it completely to them. The reason is that His superior purpose was to get them to learn that He was always in control even when things were looking bleak to them because they were in captivity, exiled in Babylon. Jeremiah 29 verse 11 in particular states: *"For I know the thoughts that I think toward you, says the Lord, thoughts of peace and not of evil, to give you a future and a hope."* This statement by the prophetic voice of the Lord was making a promise to the people and nation of Israel that even though things did not make sense at the time, God was and still is, in current times, firmly and perpetually in control of the plan He has set out for them and their future. The call was thus to them to remain hopeful of the goodness of God and His intention to bring them into a future experience of peace and not evil. The people had to depend on God, whether or not they could understand His plan and deeds.

Secondly, the scripture is a reminder that even though the people of Israel, and for that matter believers in this age, will face difficulties in life, they must always remember that God's promises are still true and certain, and therefore He must be believed and trusted completely. This must be without any strife or insistence on understanding what God is doing. As Fidelis of Sigmaringen puts it *"It is because of faith that we exchange the present for the future."* My learning actually includes the fact that our faith in the future must consistently make us choose to believe in the future of things which we do not know or even understand, because the Lord God says they are. The reality is that we might never understand that future, yet it is God's plan for us, and therefore it is enough for us to believe in it as our guaranteed future.

Another thing I have gained from listening to the Holy Spirit on this subject is His clear voice and teaching in **Hebrews 11:1-3.** *"Now faith is the substance of things hoped for, the evidence of things not seen. For by it the elders obtained a good testimony. By faith we understand that the worlds were framed by the word of God, so that the things which are seen were not made of things which are visible"*. I know we can often accept God's will when we can understand it. But He calls us further. He says we must accept it even when we are confused by it. His reason is that it is a matter of trust in His goodness, and not our understanding of our circumstances. He says when we rely on Him, we can expect Him to work miraculously in us, and then bring us an understanding of His purpose for us.

I am pleased to share at this point some of the important lessons I have received from the Holy Spirit through my periodic meditation on Hebrews 11. First, I understand now that faith is actually evidence of the spiritual world and the order of things as God has set them out to be unfolded through time. As I have said above, the Holy Spirit calls us out of our minds and imaginations to see through God's eyes the things He has set in motion in the invisible or unseen world. This is because He wants us to have the capacity to bring them into being in the visible, seen world. I fully agree now that our faith in God demands that we trust fully in Him, rely completely on His promises and cling totally to Him as our Rock of Ages.

Second, faith is a firm persuasion and expectation that God will perform all that He has promised to us in Jesus Christ. But what I have understood is that faith calls for our responsiveness, courage and sacrifices in uncertainties and challenging situations. To me, that means that for our faith to transcend the present and capture the future, we must position ourselves to receive God's promises and enforce His justice. This is only possible when we find or get to know those promises, which are so abundantly recorded in God's word, the Bible. When we know the word of promise and believe in it, we can endure the difficulties of the present and anticipate the triumphs of the future. That is faith, the one described in Hebrews 11:3.

Third, we must build on our faith and grow in it (Jude 20). This is how we can get God to manifest His power in our lives, and enable us to cope with all types of crisis, suffering, distress and anxiety. Whether we see what the future holds or not, we must prepare for it by growing in faith. That way, we are able to welcome the future and whatever comes with it as the gift of God. That is when we will begin to realize or experience the plan/thoughts of good, peace, hope and future Jeremiah 29:11 tells us about.

I am very encouraged and inspired these days when I think about the future of my son and his peers. Thoughts about their future are no more 'the avoidable things' for me. This is because like Nick Vujicic, I am no longer looking at those autistic children according to what they lack. I look at them as people who can do anything they choose to do. Their setbacks and the challenges of autism are not enough to deny them of the probable and absolute possibilities God has placed in the future ahead of them. I have just decided to have faith in that future for them. I am no longer being stressed about when those possibilities will happen. I admit I sometimes wonder what good could possibly come out of them all. But I also have something powerful in my thoughts and vision of the future, and that is the faith which says that even tragedies can turn into triumphs (**1 John 5:4**). In concluding, I urge you not to suffer and question God's goodness anymore. Rather, we must deliberately and constructively consider how His power might be made known in our trials. We must redirect our prayers not to improve our situation, but to have whatever be our circumstances demonstrate His glory.

SUFFICIENT GRACE

Nyame Adom

*__2 Corinthians 12:8-10__ reads "Concerning this thing I
pleaded with the Lord three times that it might depart
from me. And He said to me, 'My grace is sufficient
for you, for My strength is made perfect in weakness'.
Therefore most gladly I will rather boast in my
infirmities, that the power of Christ may rest upon me.
Therefore I take pleasure in infirmities, in reproaches,
in needs, in persecutions, in distresses, for Christ's
sake. For when I am weak, then I am strong."*

Paul talks of a bothersome problem about which
he prayed, but God refused to remove it. Instead,
God provided Paul sufficient grace to deal with
it. Sometimes it is tempting. We worry about how we
will make it through the days, weeks, months and years
to come. But God provides grace at the exact time we
need it. That is what we must be confident in, that God
provides His grace at the right and exact time we need it.
Our response to this must be trust.

My son Yooku has largely been a healthy and strong
child. Through his childhood to the early teen years,
he did not struggle with sicknesses nor suffer from any

particular health challenge. He is also generally not unwilling to take his medication, and so he has grown up nicely, and we are very grateful to the good Lord for that. He appeared to love his school settings, right from his toddler days. When we moved him to the Centre where he gets special needs training, he loved the environment, the training schedule and curriculum as well as the people. Before long he had made good friends, and it was obvious that he was developing new learning skills and capability to learn consistently. We were even more hopeful and encouraged when he was introduced to an inclusive classroom program, by which he spent three days of the week in mainstream classroom with kids about two grades below his age, and thus started learning basic numeracy and literacy as in regular primary school. Within those two years, and up till about age eight, he was also seeing a speech therapist once a week to help him begin to sputter out a few words, at least upon repeated promptings and expert guidance from an acclaimed professional in town. We kept our routines for hearing and speech assessments, and were comforted that there were no recommendations for hearing aids nor surgical remedies to free his vocal system to function. The expectation was that he would continue to learn to speak, write, draw and so forth like any other infant in school, albeit delayed and at a rather slow pace. But that was not to be.

Along the way and rather suddenly, Yooku lost everything verbal he had progressively learnt. He could no more even mutter audible sounds. All he was left with was a humming sound in response to anyone's prompt to speak, or sometimes in an attempt to sing to himself. He also lost interest in writing, drawing, adding on or any form of progressive play. I did some research on these developments and other things I was observing with my son. Some findings I read suggested that "autism has no cure, very little treatment and virtually no hope". The literature available seems to conclude that children with ASD have diminished psychological self-knowledge. This causes impaired memory and difficulty in remembering events. In a study by Laura Crane (2012) it was found that adults with ASD also experience reduction in recall and recovery of memory. Jones et al (2010) also found that poor social communication skills have effect on memory function, and can affect recognition of pictures, words, names and social stimuli.

This realization was devastating to me. Yes I had read quite a bit of the literature on children with autism and how they could lose their learning capabilities and regress, but I could not believe nor accept it, that it was happening to my son. I cannot explain the despair I felt. It was as though all our efforts had been wasted and grace had run out for us. I found myself asking whether one could not even thank God for the little signs of learning ability Yooku was gaining anymore, because he was fast losing them. Truly, I couldn't think straight. I used to wake up each morning dreading how I was going to pick him up after school and be told that he paid no attention or did not cooperate with his carers all day long. I wondered what the various evaluation reports given him meant, and questioned myself about all the things we as family were supposed to have done wrong for this to be happening to our child. But I also knew that we had done nothing wrong. I questioned myself why my God would look on and allow my son's destiny to look so gloomy whilst we were breaking our backs to get him into a space of possibilities, however little they may be. I was very disappointed also because this was happening soon after my son was recommended for "structured teaching". This is a disciplined work oriented and very driven program which focuses on improving a child's socialization and behavior choices. It is aimed at preparing the special needs child to move into regular classes. But as things looked at that time, he was not ready to move on and progress with that program any further.

While all this was going on, we were praying together at home one Sunday evening when my junior son suggested that we pray for Yooku to speak his few words again and resume his nice writing/copy work again. He said he just wanted his brother to be sent to the next class in his school. This was because he my junior son had been promoted to the next class both in regular school and in Sunday school, so Yooku must also go forward. This was such an encouragement and renewing strength to me. I had told myself in my personal prayer league that month that Yooku was being attacked by the enemy to challenge my faith and discourage me, and so I was asking God to fight for his cause, to protect him and favor him again. I prayed with him often in those days, laying hands on him when he retired to bed at night after his cranky night episodes. Day in and out, it was difficult to keep the peace and hope within my heart, because the signs of change I was praying for were not manifesting, and I increasingly felt he was slipping into a shut down of himself from all of us. The cry in those days was mainly "God help us", because I felt afraid to tell dear family and friends that we were losing our tangible gains from the training and teaching regimen. Personally, I was afraid to make this known, whether as a means to call for more prayer or to court empathy, so we were alone in our "little world of despair". I knew that trusting God was the thing to do, but doing it in those days seriously hanged in the balance.

Then came an episode I cherish so much now. I was out in Northern Ghana to do some work. All alone in my hotel room one night, I watched the movie 'Breakthrough'. It is based on the true story of an American teenaged boy, John Smith, who was rescued from the bottom of an icy lake. He remained unconscious for about 72 hours and was declared clinically dead by doctors. But his mother held on to his feet and prayed insistently to God for her son to come back to life. She was radical, defiant and unyielding, and John indeed woke up, back to life and lives on today. I remember I simply prayed shortly that night before I slept, asking God to bring my son's memory and learning capabilities back to him. In my mind I simply thought, if He could bring a dead boy back to life because his mother prayed, then He should at least bring my son's memory back to him. I had no struggle in my spirit saying that, and I slept quite soundly too, because I was tired from trekking all day. What I continue to cherish about that episode is that I woke up in the morning, and I literally felt as though I was being hugged by a very huge (I mean big and tall) fellow who rubbed my back. It felt so very peaceful, and the silence was truly golden.I received no direct audible message, but a renewed confidence and assurance from Him that nothing would be lost. I did not really connect that feeling and presence to my prayer. I just thanked God for the new day and peaceful assurance I had within, and went on with the mission of my trip as usual, and returned home a few days later. It was when I was completing my field report that I momentarily reflected on that experience. At that time I had not observed any change or new development in my son's situation, but I believed God would answer me, and I was content to wait for that time, even though I was equally disappointed that regression had occurred in the first place.

But my reflection on that night prayer and feeling hugged by a mighty strong fellow who also comforted me actually led me to something important and worth sharing. God uses dreams to reveal His plans and also to effect His decision about certain situations in our lives. When we pray at night before sleeping, we need to open up our hearts to Him and trust that He may choose the sleep period to give us a head-start for the new day. God uses the night to draw closures in our lives, as well as begin new developments which may be immediate or short term. He also uses some dreams to prompt us about long term plans and purposes He has for us. I believe all we need to do is to keep the memory of the dreams, pray about them and particularly stay open to the voice of the Spirit as we read portions of scripture in our normal devotions and study sessions. When a particular scripture pops up or stays stuck on your mind about the dream you had some time ago, that may be God's direct word to you to interpret the dream and to instruct or direct you further on with it.

The Holy Spirit later drew my attention to what was required of me and indeed all believers regarding certain aspects of God's grace. **2 Corinthians 12:9** speaks directly about what Paul received from the Lord as answer to his prayer and instruction for continuous living. From this scripture, it appears quite clearly that God has already determined His measure of grace for us in our situations of distress and despair. He has also perfected His strength for us in those moments of our weakness. Based on this I have gained an understanding that we must learn to recognize the persistent labor of the flesh and its interference in God's plan. We must resist the flesh when our anxiety and distress is mounting. All things that are accomplished for God, whether salvation itself or the life that follows, are accomplished by His initiative and power through our dependence and faith. It is God's predetermined act of grace that we must believe in. This life is all about Him, and so we should not stress ourselves by making it about us.

I wish to share with believers, and also encourage all who may be going through distressing situations, that we must attract the power of God to change our destinies by gladly seeing glory in the infirmities He has permitted in our lives. We must not feel punished, short-changed or even think that we have been handed a misfortune in life. Godliness with contentment is what God calls a great gain, nothing else (1 Timothy 6:6).

By a certain coincidence, I have since then read 'Glorious Intruder' a best-selling book by **Joni Eareckson Tada.** In her chapter on Grace, I read these refreshing words *"God's grace is not only adequate, it is available for every time of need. We don't have to plead for it, beg for it, or do penance to be worthy of it. No, God's grace, His love in action, is not a favour for which we must implore, it is a gift we are invited to enjoy. We don't need to ask God to make His grace sufficient for us; He has already assured us that whatever the hardship, there is an adequate compensating amount of grace ready and available for the taking. Grace has been given and it only remains for us to receive it. How wide and deep and high and long the promise of that grace really is. It is sufficient. So whatever your particular heartache or headache, approach the throne of grace with confidence so that you may find grace to help in your time of need. Drink deep of it. It's yours. And it's enough."*

Months and years on from this episode and related learning, my son has regained his memory and learning capabilities. He has gained a larger understanding and appreciation of language, his environment, relational behaviors and so forth. He is still not communicating verbally, and continues to deal with his sensory challenges, constricted attention span and delayed behavioral responses. But he is his better self than before, learning and achieving his goals and purposes at his own pace, and is very much a lovely gift from God. Every look at him and recollections from the moments and events of his life confirm to me that God has indeed provided His grace sufficiently so far, and so we can continue to trust and depend on him for the rest of the journey. From time to time, my wife and I enjoy and encourage ourselves by the wonderful Ghanaian choral music by Newlove Annan. The lyrics are a mix of Ghanaian languages and English, which collectively translate as follows:

Grace and mercy has brought me here this day

Lord God but for your grace this life would be very difficult indeed

The battle is quite fierce, yet the grace leads me on daily

Lord God it's your grace that has brought me thus far.

You never made a promise that the journey would be easy

But your grace and mercy has brought me thus far

Your grace and mercy is all I need

Your grace and mercy has brought me thus far.

We continue to live by faith and fervent expectation that God would grant us the full manifestation of His word as decreed by the Apostle Peter. ***2 Peter 1:2-4*** *says "Grace and peace be multiplied to you in the knowledge of God and of Jesus our Lord, as His divine power has given to us all things that pertain to life and godliness, through the knowledge of Him who called us by glory and virtue".*

THE POWER OF EMPATHY

Bese Saka

"Empathy is a great gift. I encourage you to practice and share it at every opportunity because it heals those who give, as well as those who receive. When you are confronted with hard times, tragedies or challenges, instead of looking inward, look to those around you. Instead of feeling wounded and seeking pity, find someone with greater wounds and help them heal. Understand that your grief or pain is legitimate, but suffering is part of the human condition, and reaching out to someone else is a way of healing yourself while helping others heal too". Nick Vujicic in Life Without Limits.

For this chapter, I pay tribute to my very good couple-folks, brothers and sisters in the faith with whom my family has shared wonderful times and moments. Ato & Loretta, Charles & Jennifer, Charles & Cynthia, Fiifi & Persis, Ben & Mercy, Theophilus & Abena, Foster & Frances, Laud & Hilda, Nana & Vivian, Frank & Louisa, Victor & Andrea are all high school and college mates of my wife and I. We are now colleagues in a family life fellowship. Our original ties and bonds begun in our long lasting commitments to youth evangelism, which brought us together in our days in high schools in different parts of Ghana. I wish to particularly thank them all for standing with us in prayer. Collectively, these folks have and continue to lift up prayer for our Yooku and us, Tuesday after Tuesday, asking and trusting God to heal him completely from everything limiting and disabling in his life due to autism. They have prayed and stood firm on the promise that God answers prayer in His wise timing. We bless the Lord for the many answers to prayer, and remain grateful to each one of them for their empathy and sacrifices.

I have had certain experiences and learning that illustrate the fact that there is so much power in empathy. It is important that we consciously make choices to empathize with ordinary non-professional people and even families who battle with things like parenting difficult and wayward children, caring for persons with different disabilities, raising children with developmental difficulties/challenges and several other stressful human conditions. What really is this empathy? I understand it to mean the ability to emotionally appreciate and share the feelings of others, such that they do not see themselves as burdened and all alone. It involves actions that show that one has an understanding or awareness, or sensitivity to vicariously experience the feelings, thoughts and circumstances of others.

People sometimes do not recognize that children with autism are very unpredictable and largely irregular in their behavior. For this reason, parents and guardians of these children easily get misunderstood, mistreated and sometimes accused of failing to raise their children properly and keep them disciplined. Our society is not well exposed to autism as a challenging developmental condition. Public awareness of the condition is very low, and for that reason autistic children do not have any special treatment as people with different abilities. Autistic persons elsewhere are provided for such that they do not have to wait in queues in places like hospitals and malls or shopping centers. There are places where autistic children for instance can communicate effectively with gadgets and sign language such that they can get by in schools, playgrounds and in places of worship. There are facilities for their use on buses and trains, in gymnasia and libraries for instance in developed countries which do not exist in our society. Because of this context, raising an autistic child in our society places one in an "all eyes on me" situation. This is what, in my humble view, creates an extraordinary need for and benefits from empathy for persons and families with children who have different forms of disabilities.

Generally, people need empathy from others, from neighbors, colleagues and superiors, and from relations and even partners some of the time. But it appears autistic persons and disabled children in particular need empathy all the time. I dare say their parents, guardians and carers may also need such empathy as well. This is because autistic children often settle on certain routines. People who raise and train them tend to program them to go through those routines, and so a question of uncertainty arises when they are seen deviating from their fixated routines. That change leaves the children unstable and their parents/carers confused. The disturbing outcome is that the children may throw tantrums, become uncooperative or even stage a shutdown, which in turn attracts the shun and scorn of society.

In my humble view, and judging from my personal experience, empathy is the singular powerful social response that makes the emotional and psychological imbalances autistic behavior creates less burdensome for both the person with autism and the parent or care-giver. When children and adult persons living with autism engage in disruptive and sometimes disgusting behaviors, they need empathy to help them calm down and get well composed again. At the same time their parents and relations also need empathy to enable them properly overcome the shame and scorn they fall into within society. It has been my practice to pray for the children and parents I come across in the social circles of autism in my country for quite a while. We all need the blessing of empathy from the Lord and our society at large. The power of empathy is seen when the parents network shares information for solving problems with their children, their orientation and other support systems they live by. Through prayer and reading the scriptures, I have learnt how to show empathy, encouragement and support particularly to parents in my network, and have gained some knowledge and guidance which I share below.

Romans 5:5 *reads "And hope makes not ashamed, because the love of God is shed abroad in our hearts by the Holy Spirit, which is given unto us".*

Paul suggests through this verse of scripture that Christians and people with express faith in Jesus Christ should live with a hope that is not aligned to the observable and physical developments or achievement of goals in their lives, but one focused on the unfailing word of God that He is trustworthy and gracious in His promises. In Paul's view, Christians should see suffering of all sorts as part of God's recipe for our growth. The challenges that confront our individual lives are meant to exact total dependence on God from us. He thus admonishes us not to be ashamed when the physical realities of our lives appear to be contrary to the expectations of our hope.

We must learn from this scripture that God has shown us so much empathy Himself, and so we must hold very high our hope in Him without making any room for shame and disappointment. This is the truth, whether or not we see certain desired changes. God has done this by placing His Holy Spirit in our hearts to bear the fruit of love, patience and long suffering (James 1:2-5). We must receive and embrace the Holy Spirit and the love in Him. Maintaining our hope and trust in God regardless of our current/immediate circumstances is the highest expression of glorifying Him, and it must be our preferred response to His giving us His Son as well as His Spirit to dwell within us (John 1:14). The author of the Book of Hebrews confirms this in **Hebrews 4:15-16**, which reads

"For we do not have a High Priest who cannot sympathize with our weaknesses, but was in all points tempted as we are, yet without sin. Let us therefore come boldly to the

throne of grace, that we may obtain mercy and find grace to help in time of need".

This clearly shows us that we can rely on the empathy of our Lord Himself as we struggle with whatever difficult situations in our lives, and also go to Him in prayer to obtain His mercy and grace to enable us cope. This has been a great encouragement to me, and gives me every reason to remain hopeful for the breakthroughs and good future I am trusting and praying for in my son's life, and in each of his peers living with autism.

A few years ago I noticed and understood something wonderful about empathetic prayer which has continued to assure me that God is always on our case and responds appropriately when we intercede in prayer for others and vice versa. The Book of Daniel reveals in chapter 2 the troubles of the all powerful King Nebuchadnezzar of ancient Babylon. He is said to have have had a dream that left him with a troubled spirit, sleeplessness and anxiety. This brought about a threat of death on Daniel's life and that of several other prophets and the heathen magicians in the land. They were to die if they failed to tell and interpret the dream the king had. But the significant thing is that, Daniel went home and got his companions into prayer, seeking God's revelation of the secret of the king's dream. From **Daniel 2:17-23** we learn about how God intervened and made Daniel great before the king and the entire generation in Babylon by giving him understanding (unction) to handle the confusion and anxiety. It all came about when the friends of Daniel gathered to pray in empathy and in solidarity with him at the time of crisis. Everything changed when Daniel's friends prayed for him about his precarious situation.

The greatest thing a person can do for another is to pray for him. In other words, to speak to God on behalf of man is the highest service one can render. This is so powerful, because the devil attacks people and leaves them stressed and confused, just so that they cannot pray. So to pray for such people is to take away the stress and confusion. As I have said earlier, the intercessory prayer of my brethren is an act of empathy which has enabled my family and I go through so many rough times. I know this because we have had very bad episodes with Yooku which I believe were miraculously healed when they prayed. I have shared above some episodes of biting people and biting themselves when some autistic children feel stressed. But there have also been days of repeated head-butting, screaming loudly and smashing glass windows in my home. Only God knows how my son remained safe before and until we were able to restrain him by tying him up, arms and legs in ropes. The little bruises and swollen flesh, in my view, did not match the destruction caused and the energy expended in doing so. But somehow he survived, many thanks to God.

Some nights have been unique for my son for the reason that the regular sleeping pills had zero effect, and so sleep was replaced with sometimes hours of slapping walls and banging doors. On two occasions when I called on my brethren to remember us in prayer and intercede for a calming spirit upon my son, the knack for biting left him, and the heightened sleeplessness left him alone too. I have lived it, and I believe it, that the Holy Spirit still responds and answers us when we intercede, standing in empathy for fellow sufferers in the faith as we battle the issues of our lives. It is said that the devil smiles when we plan to pray. Then he laughs when we get too busy to pray. He trembles when we actually pray, but he dreads it when we stand together in fervent prayer. We must therefore encourage ourselves to pray continually, remembering that it is God who answers prayer, and He has promised to answer in the best way to every prayer.

My further learning from the Holy Spirit which I want to share so that believers can activate and benefit from the power of empathy from the Lord and well meaning people is this. Firstly, *recognize* that the Holy Spirit is within you, and allow Him to lead you into all truth. Do not be anxious and be driven by your feelings when you are thrown into confusion by the disruptions that come into your life. The Holy Spirit within you is always ready to lead you in moments when you are overwhelmed by shame and distress, and He does that with utmost empathy, because He is familiar with all our weaknesses. Secondly, *rely on* the Holy Spirit to give you victory over every temptation and doubt from the devil about the hope and expectation you have in the Lord. Long for and pray for anything that is God's will for you without doubting, and He will work out the miracles of your life in its time. Thirdly, *reach out* to your brethren and neighbors with your acts of kindness and acceptance, and do not hold back no matter your challenging situations. As Nick has stated above, when confronted with hardship, tragedies and challenges, reaching out to someone else is a way of healing yourself while helping others heal too. I believe this is in the nature (although in indirect context) of what the Apostle Paul illustrated to the faithful brethren in Colosse as stated in **Colossians 1:9-13** that *"for this reason we also, since the day we heard it, do not cease to pray for you, and to ask that you may be filled with the knowledge of His will in all wisdom and spiritual understanding. That you may walk worthy of the Lord, fully pleasing to Him, being fruitful in every good work and increasing in the knowledge of God, strengthened with all might according to His glorious power, for all patience and longsuffering with joy, giving thanks to the Father who has qualified us to be partakers of the inheritance of the saints in the light. He has delivered us from the power of darkness and conveyed us into the kingdom of the Son of His love"*.

Reading from **"Clippings From My Notebook"**, I found this prayer which was said by Corrie ten Boom in gratitude for Romans 5:5 which I have quoted above. She said "Thank You Lord Jesus, that You have brought into my heart the love of God through the Holy Spirit, who is given to me. Thank You Father, that Your love in me is victorious over the bitterness in me and cruelty around me". I say Amen to that.

In concluding this chapter, I wish to ask you to learn to pray that prayer, because you have a great task to overcome the challenges and tragedies you will face in your life as a representative of the Lord Jesus Christ. If you permit the Holy Spirit given to you in your heart, He will work through you and make you victorious in the battles of your life.

THE LORD WILL BUILD FOR THEM

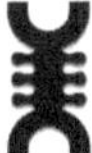

Osiadan Nyame

My tribute for this chapter goes to Mrs Serwah Quaynor, the Founder and Executive Director of Autism Awareness Care & Training Centre (AACT) in Accra. I have chosen to thank Auntie Serwah for maintaining the hope and resilient faith in the belief that because children with autism are special children of the Lord, He will build a place (centre) for them. I recall that in my conversations with her on the subject, I have counted not less than ten times when she had said, "the Lord will build for them a centre". She somehow saw within her inner self a beautiful and convenient centre built by the Lord Himself for His children. She kept saying this when we were struggling with all the ideas of finding land within the city, raising sponsorship and the needed financial resources to build a permanent centre with facilities fit for children with autism. Today, that hope and faith in the Lord has borne its fruit, and our children are the better for it.

Children with autism in Ghana do not have many options by way of available centres and schools for special education in which they can access the special-purpose creative curricula suitable for them. There are only a few schools/centres that run special education programmes for children with disabilities. However, it appears much of the emphasis in terms of national policies and public infrastructure is placed on visually impaired, hearing impaired and physically challenged children. Not much provision is made for children with autism spectrum disorder (ASD), cerebral palsy (CP) and the like. The available schools/centres around the country that provide care, training and education for children with autism in particular are all private institutions with very scanty functional facilities required for their skills development and integration into society as they grow. This is quite unfortunate as children with autism have several learning difficulties and therefore deserve much more policy attention and infrastructural provisions from the State.

AACT is a private charitable institution providing a range of educational and social support services for children with autism and their families. There is virtually no public/state support for this and the other schools set up to train and educate children with disabilities like CP and Asperger's syndrome. Founders and directors/trustees/ managers of such institutions have to create and develop almost all the infrastructure needed for the training and education of these special needs children. That is very expensive, and they cannot easily raise funding or even credit for such. This situation leaves them not sufficiently resourced and equipped to run the appropriate curriculum, and therefore some of the children may end up not being able to develop their innate skills and full potential. This had been a challenge AACT grappled with for years, and my association with Mrs. Quaynor revealed to me how burdensome it is to find the right support and financing resources to build and develop anything for such institutions. This is because in the Ghanaian society, people often think of charitable acts as giving and providing little food items and other simple consumables to needy, vulnerable and less privileged persons and institutions. Even the corporate institutions and benevolent organizations do not easily nor regularly support the perhaps marginalized groups in society like children with disabilities, even though they very well could undertake developmental projects for them as their corporate social responsibility. The impression one gets when engaging leaders of corporates and some social clubs and societies of repute to consider sponsoring projects or supporting institutions catering for children with disabilities is that they are somewhat forgotten about by the larger society in the various schemes of planning and development initiatives. This is quite sad, because it is widespread and difficult to change.

Our breakthrough came when in 2018, My Sisters Keepers Organization decided to commit funds they raised from a gala to support the work of AACT. We met as Board of Trustees of AACT to discuss with them the needs of AACT and what options of activities and projects we could commit the funds to. Renovating the rented premises where the centre was located then appeared acceptable to the Sisters, who by this time had begun seeing themselves as sponsors of AACT. I was opposed to the idea of the renovation, because I thought the premises was already small for the number of students and thus the need to relocate was overdue. But I also did not know or could not guess how much funds was available to be spent, so I did not speak of what I thought was the better option. In that meeting, I knew that the better option was to ask them to sponsor the building (development) of a new centre, designed and built for the specific purposes of the training and education of the children, but I did not raise it. Thankfully, the meeting ended without a concrete decision. We agreed to have some costing and budgeting done for renovating the centre as well as for procuring certain equipment for use by the students, and the decisions were deferred till another meeting within a month from then. That gave me an opportunity to pray fervently asking God specifically to make the request of supporting the building of an entirely new ultra-modern centre with facilities for the special needs of the children acceptable to the sisters. Before long, I had the inner conviction that the sisters could help to build the new centre. I prayed specifically for that and the wisdom to convince the Board members that we should request for that.

I met Mrs Quaynor at the centre, and we discussed how to go about this. As usual, she shared with me her strong faith in the belief that God would build the centre miraculously for the children. This time round, I asked her what she expected from the ball and how we could encourage the sisters to do something else to raise more funds for the building in case they were focused only on a quick donation and not a growing collaboration. Honestly, I expected her to say something like "my instinct tells me so and so" or "I don't even know how much was raised at the ball" or "let's see what God will do". But guess what, she just said, I know the song that says "God is Working". I knew the song too, so we naturally started singing it together. This song, recorded by Brooklyn Tabernacle Choir, has the following lyrics:

God is working
He's still working
God is working even now
Though we often don't know just how
God is working
He's still working
God is working even now.
Though you cannot see
And you can't quite understand
Remember God is still in control
He has promised to bring you through somehow
And He's working even now.
Hallelujah
He's working even now
Hallelujah
He's working even now
Though we often don't know just how

God is working
He's still working
God is working even now.
God is working
He is working Even now
God is working
Even right now.

After the encouraging fun of singing this song, we continued chatting about the strategy to use to get the needed support for building the new centre. This was after we had spent about three years frantically seeking corporate sponsorship for this goal of a new centre and failed woefully. All we could say for the effort at that time was that two individuals had maintained their commitment to pay the rent for the premises year after year for five years. Mrs Quaynor lamented how stressful and sometimes painful it had been when well to do people in society, and obviously successful companies had turned down humble requests from AACT for support to implement developmental projects including procurement of skills training equipment and the building of a new centre. She recounted the unfortunate view some people have that supporting children with autism was humanitarian alright, but did not really hold any prospects because to them those children are unteachable and therefore would achieve nothing from the investment. I also remembered how often my meeting to discuss proposals and requests from AACT with the managers and owners of some businesses to support the children ended in very disappointing ways.

We shared a common pain about the lack of interest by the government of our country in the development of special education systems and institutions, as well as the general despondency of corporate bodies in our society to facilitate the training of autistic children through charitable donations. In the end, we had to encourage ourselves to continue trusting God to show His children His own uncommon favor. Meanwhile, we agreed to change the discussions with the sisters in our next meeting from spending the funds on renovating the rented premises to building a new centre. The Quaynor family graciously donated a parcel of land within the city of Accra for the new centre to be developed thereon.

Praying for this dream of a new centre for AACT was an urgent matter for me, and I had to involve my family to do intense intercession before the Lord for this. I remember how I would go to the Lord in prayer, reminding Him of how He enabled Nehemiah mobilize the people to rebuild the broken walls of Jerusalem, and Zerubbabel and Joshua to build the house of the Lord (see Haggai 1:14-15). A few days later, I went again to Mrs Quaynor and asked that we make more direct our request to the sisters by describing the sort of building and facilities we desired to be included in the new centre. It was all to enable us to be more convincing and to share the vision and passion to see it done with them. We had a team of four put together the details of the new building, which I composed into a brief for the architect and engineers who would design the project to use. Praying for this project by this time was shared with the staff and parents, and we were all encouraged to ask God to build for His children a new centre by Mrs Quaynor.

When the next meeting with the sisters was held, it was agreed that the funds and additional efforts be put to building a new centre as that was the real need. The sisters quickly arranged a meeting with an estate developer and the brief was discussed and accepted as well. The envisioned centre was suddenly coming into being. God was working it out, the help had come, and the faith, that is the substance of the building hoped for was to become the reality. Along the way, the Quaynor and Beng Asare familes also graciously donated additional funds to help complete the final finishing works on the building and render it ready for use. I was very happy that this was happening, and remain grateful that it has been completed for the use of the children. The first phase of the new centre, which is actually the ground floor of the designed 2-storey building was actually handed over to AACT to operate in June 2020.

I have learnt from this encounter certain profound things from the Holy Spirit about trusting Him with our needs. I now proceed to share a few of them from the scriptures with you. We often approach certain needs of ours as though God is depending on us to do the work while He supports us in the background. But as I reflected on what God has done regarding the new centre for AACT, the Holy Spirit taught me that we must always depend on God to do the work while we are behind the scenes believing in

Him and moving at His command. We must be quick to believe and hesitant to interfere in the work of grace He is doing in our lives. In the verses of **Psalm 118**, the author celebrates the goodness, deliverance and provision of the Lord with thanksgiving and praise. The admissions and professions of the author suggest to us that we should see all the achievements and developments in our lives as the works of God done to show His omnipotence, mercy and wisdom.

Psalm 127:1 reads, *"Unless the Lord builds the house, they labor in vain who build it. Unless the Lord guards the city, the watchman stays awake in vain"*. I have learnt from reflecting on this verse that even though humans desiring to develop think they must labor and apply their skills and resources to achieve their goals, God remains eternally in control of all successes and failures we encounter. Thus without God, we can do nothing.

Hebrews 3:4 also reads, *"For every house is built by someone, but He who built all things is God"*. This means we must never forget that God has a plan for everything and ultimately builds everything. As the Creator of all things, He gives us the opportunity to mobilize and implement things He has set up as missions for us, but we must know that whatever we achieve is only a small part of His grand plan. We must always be driven by what we believe and pray to God for, especially what is within His word and will for us. We should never be driven by what we have or can afford. Once what we desire to achieve is right and glorifying to God, we must focus on what God can do and not on our lack of resources, imaginations, stress or even failures in the past. Jesus Christ demonstrated to us the right attitude we must adopt in our race of faith before God.

In **Hebrews 12:1-2**, we read this, *"therefore we also, since we are surrounded by so great a cloud of witnesses, let us lay aside every weight and sin which so easily ensnares us, and let us run with endurance the race that is set before us, looking unto Jesus, the author and finisher of our faith, who for the joy that was set before Him endured the cross, despising the shame, and has sat down at the right hand of the throne of God"*.

When we focus on what God can do, we get to see His 'To Do list', and thus get to know where to go, whom to go to, when to go and how to get there on time. We therefore do not continue to struggle in our efforts to mobilize and apply God's resources to implement His plan. That is why when God says He makes all things beautiful in its time (Ecclesiastes 3:11), we can rely on it as the truth and foundation of our abiding hope in Him. The times and seasons for planting and harvesting reveal to us that God has a plan and order in sequence for everything. The cycle of life demands that we focus completely on God and run the race of faith without losing hope. If we wait patiently for God in our pursuit of His will for us, we can count on His faithfulness in unfolding His plan, and we will have our needs met beautifully in its time.

GRATEFUL HEARTS

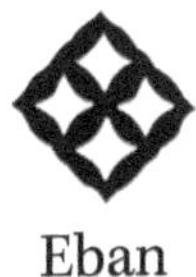

Eban

This chapter is dedicated to Corrie ten Boom of blessed memory, my remote mentor and grandmother in the faith. I never met this woman in person before she passed on to glory, but my reading of her publications has made a most significant impact on my view of how detailed the interests of God are in the lives of committed believers in this age.

For over a decade I have been taking my son each morning to school. For this reason I have met with and have a personal relationship with some of the children in the school. I get to engage them, play with some of them sometimes, and have a special friendship with at least three of them. These children can be so warm, and yet other times they can be very aggressive, disruptive and destructive. I have thus learnt to manage their moods and postures, and continue to find out how best to cope with them. However, I would admit any day that no two autistic children are predictably the same.

Arnold was about eight years old when I met him and started almost a daily interaction with him. He is in his late teens now. He has a few spoken words and thus can be classified as verbal. But he doesn't always make coherent speech, because he says things which are not consistently conversational. But for an autistic person, he is doing well with those few words and sentences with which he expresses himself. Arnold is my friend. He comes over to me whenever I get to the compound of his school, and calls me "Daddy how are you?". For him, as soon as I appear in the morning, the natural thing after calling out my name as stated above is to say to me "I am fine". When I appear in the afternoon or evening after school, the natural statement to me is "Yooku is going home". All I have to do is to respond to him in the words "Thank you Arnold". If I should fail or refuse to say so, I would be in all manner of trouble. What do I mean? If I don't say "Thank you Arnold", then anything among these would be happening to me without fail. He may be banging on the bonnet of my car, spinning around me to frustrate me from moving/walking around, slapping me on the back or dragging me by the hand. I just have to say "Thank you Arnold" to be free, and trust you me I am always instantly free once I say so. There is virtually no more conversation or interaction beyond this. So the routine of friendship between "my son Arnold" and I is just to exchange those three sentences between us. I will tell you about the gratitude I get for that shortly.

Irene is just about ten years old. She is also my special friend, because she is the self- appointed receptionist for parents who bring her mates to their school. She has a way of waiting at the entrance, and once you bring your ward, she would grab your hand and drag you to the office to greet the administrator. Irene has no speech, but she would so nicely bow to courtesy as a well-groomed girl should greet. I guess she says to herself in her mind that she is greeting the administrator for the parent. Once she is acknowledged as having come to greet, she happily leaves the parent alone and goes to wait for the next person. I am told she does that for about six parents each morning before she goes to settle in her classroom. I guess again that she probably considers her self-given social duty done for the morning, and then retires to the classroom to learn for the day. My special deal of gratitude with Irene would also be shared shortly below.

Joshua is the other special kiddy-friend I have at the Autism Centre. Handsome and athletic Joshua sees it as a must to say "Good Morning" to me. He then would ask "How are you", and once I answer him as being fine, I get a hand-clap from him as reward. You should see the joy with which he would run off to do whatever else he has to do that morning once he has greeted and clapped for me. Joshua knows no other period of the day. It is good morning all the time once he has seen me, his friend. I know he greets several other persons, including some of his trainers the same way.

I have also noticed Sena, another happy little girl whose business is to hug all her female carers when she comes to school in the morning. Sena has no speech, and so I guess hugging is her way of greeting and welcoming herself to school. It is compulsory for the lady carers to hug her, because if you fail to do so she would follow you around the compound until you hug her. They have all learnt their lesson from Sena, and she gets along well with them when they obey her command.

There is also Nana Sakyi, a gentle lad who is noted for his insistent finger snapping with others. Once he notices you, he would walk up to you, shake hands and snap your finger. If you don't know about that and therefore refuse to heed, you would not be free from him until you have allowed him to do so. For first time acquaintances, he can actually drag his colleague to you and demonstrate it to you, so you would also allow him to do so to you before you can be free.

Such acts and mannerisms as described above are the fixations of these children with autism. It is quite difficult to understand how these acts so much satisfy and appease them so that they can relax and function well just after doing so. I have accepted it that some personality needs get satisfied when these children get to act out their "manners and gestures", and so people who know and can associate them with such gestures should accept them as well and make them feel all the more welcome within their social circles.

But there are thoughts and ideas that these children and their acts have brought to me personally which I consider worth sharing. Apart from learning to accept them for their personality differences, I have observed and seen what I like to call their personal and spiritual gratitude. **When I look beyond the struggles of these and other children with autism I have encountered, and into**

their sacred beings, I see that theirs are truly 'grateful hearts' indeed. They struggle so much to express or put across their requests and desires, and yet they settle in to such peace with themselves once they have been accepted or responded to appropriately. It is beautiful how they wave at you, bid you good-bye or smile at you when they know you have been friendly to them that morning or day.

I wish I had a succinct way of advocating for all people to accept their friendship and graciously respond to them rather than ignore or avoid them. Arnold for instance does have his mood swings as a typical autistic person, but I am grateful and can say quite confidently that he is faithful in coming to me to act out his routines in the morning or after school. I don't know and probably cannot know by scientific exactitude, but I believe he comes to me to say his few words or act out his protest because he has a grateful heart for his friend in me, and strives to keep that friend. I believe Joshua is grateful for people who respond to his greeting, and is eager to give his little gift of appreciation in his routine of clapping for them. These children are not babies. They act out their routines on purpose, and are calculated in the responses they expect or require from others. For this reason, I suspect they are grateful for the positive responses and sad when they are ignored and rejected. This may be the norm for most persons, but I also think that as the theory on autistic sensitivity says, their heightened needs for acceptance also breeds deep sorrow and a sense of rejection which makes them recoil and shut down.

I remember praying for them one Saturday night as I went walking with my son. My prayer was that God would make me and other parents grateful for these children, so that we would receive His strength and wisdom to enable us guide and give them our best support. I was praying that way because there were times in those days when it was so tiring keeping up with my son and yet seeing virtually no progress. This was just after I had agreed with the speech therapist he was seeing to go off the weekly schedule. We agreed because the speech would just not come, and he still has no speech yet. What happened? Nothing. But days later, I went to the school and just when I drove in I felt an inner urge to look at the children. I looked at them in their usual ways about the compound, left my son and went away. I was quite disappointed I did not observe anything spectacular looking at them, so I just went on my way. Then the notable thing happened. A friend forwarded to me a poster around lunchtime via Whatsapp of **1 Corinthians 13:12-13.** This is what this passage of scripture says in the New Living Translation, *"For now we see things imperfectly as in a cloudy mirror, but then we will see everything with perfect clarity. All that I know now is partial and incomplete, but then I will know everything completely, just as God now knows me completely. Three things will last forever, faith, hope and love, and the greatest of these is love".*

I paid attention to these two verses and have continued to think about what it says since then. In the context of the children I had to look at before this word came to me, I believe I have received some measure of increase in all three elements of the fruit of the Spirit mentioned. I am confident that my faith in God for a better future for them is intact and growing. I am also hopeful that they will do well and have something purposeful to do in life as they grow up. And in addition I see myself loving them day by day, with or without their unusual manners, and it seems to come easily to me now. But as said earlier, I have continued to pray and look out for insights from scripture and the Holy Spirit how best to love and support these children to find and realize their purpose. Thankfully I have found some perspectives from Corrie ten Boom.

According to Tante Corrie, *"the love of God is a protection as well as a weapon. It guards us against impatience, against zeal without sense, against annoyance, against bitterness, against gloating. This love knows no limit to its endurance, no end to its trust, no fading of its hope, it can outstand anything. It is, in fact, the one thing that still stands when all else has fallen"*.

I have pondered over this for a while. She was thinking and discussing the love of God for humankind as set out in **Romans 5:5**. But at the same time I find the statement as an apt direction and guidance for me and other parents who may be praying for the strength to keep going on with supporting their children with autism. The statement, when further elucidated shows quite clearly how everyone who bears up another person (such as a child with autism) with the love of God would become enabled by the Holy Spirit to:

a) protect that person from physical dangers and spiritual attacks

b) fight for him/her and pursue their interests as much as possible

c) live patiently with them

d) encourage or tolerate them to grow at their own pace of progress

I understand from the statement that God's love would enable one to contain all the annoyance that autistic persons can create, and help to overcome any form of bitterness and gloating. What I find most comforting is the view that this love endures without limits and remains trusting all the time. Without any doubt, this is what we need, and I cannot agree more that it is only this love that can keep us standing throughout the trials of living with autism and remain grateful.

Furthermore, I have sought to consciously practice what Corrie ten Boom states above, particularly because I want to permanently overcome impatience, zeal without sense, annoyance and bitterness, just as she puts it. I must say it is a difficult task, but also a very rewarding one. It is refreshing to walk away knowing that you spent two minutes to be a friend and make that yearning little child happy. For them, the little responses to their gestures bring so much comfort and happiness, and they are able to settle within themselves the heightened desire for acceptance. According to William Stillman, the sense of acceptance and assurance of safety that an autistic person can derive from a known friend is most effective in calming down the sensory tensions they suffer from just before their meltdowns. The feeling of visible appreciation and praise also helps them overcome their anxieties.

I am convinced the children I am talking about here have grateful hearts. Therefore I urge my readers to open up to all children with autism, accommodate and accept them with all their differences. That is sure to make a big difference in their socialization and self-worth, though unspoken. To my dear parents of children with autism, I encourage you to accept it that some things happen to us from which we never recover, and they disrupt the normalcy of our lives. Some may say that is how life is. However, I urge us all to always look at our extraordinary children and re-echo to ourselves the profound mantra by Kerry Magro, that "AUTISM DOESN'T COME WITH AN INSTRUCTION GUIDE. IT COMES WITH A FAMILY WHO WILL NEVER GIVE UP". We who live it know that "autism is nothing but hardwork". Perhaps unlike several other ventures in this life, I dare say there are no guarantees of expected breakthroughs for every child with autism in terms of the set goals for raising and training them. But certainly, there are rewards for every effort that is made.

EPILOGUE

I am so thankful that you have stayed with me throughout this book. My prayer is for you to gain an understanding of God's presence and interest in everything that happens to you in life. In these 12 Dates I have shared some experiences and lessons, both from the manifestations of autism and the insightful teaching of the Holy Spirit. Many benefits can be derived from practising the guiding principles and activating the elements of faith set out herein. As part of my final words, I have chosen to point to certain cultural symbols of the Akan peoples of Ghana which I have used as highlighting icons for the chapters. They are to serve as an inspirational aid to enable you remain steadfast in your battles with autism reflected in each chapter. This is because much of the societal failure to accept the differences of persons with autism and support them both spiritually and physically to realize their potentials is borne out of misunderstanding of cultural heritage and secularism. I must hasten to add though that there is also the rejection fueled by ignorance and poverty.

Notions of secularization continue to push believers into the margins of life. In the name of human rights and modernism, families must be encouraged to stand up for the benefits of their children with autism. We must emphasise the elements of our Christian beliefs such as healing and miracles, hope in the future, trust in divine purposes and faith in God. But in certain parts of the world, cultural beliefs are sources of the standards and rules used to deny children with autism and other disorders the appropriate socialization and training support. The use of these few symbols is to demonstrate that within the varied notions of human religious, cultural and secularist orientations in our societies, there is room for acceptance and support for differences and human weaknesses where diligent search is made for common good.

These heritage signs connote ideals which align with the shared experiences and lessons discussed in this book. They are chosen to highlight the chapters and to show that within our cultural context, there are aspirations which reinforce the need to make room for human differences and weaknesses in the interest of social cohesion and fulfilment of positive divine obligations. An understanding of these symbolic icons will help eschew rejection and denial of the weak and disabled in our societies, and rather create acceptance and support systems for them. We must remember and instinctively adopt the teaching of the Holy Spirit in relation to our dependence on God, the benevolence of God, the obligation to have faith in God and trust Him with all our challenges, and our common duty to love and support one another, especially the weak, vulnerable and disabled.

The symbol called **"Ohene Aniwa"** which means "God (Eternal King) is all knowing and all seeing" highlights Chapter One. The import is that we must remember that God sees each of us as we go through the varied challenges frustrating our good lives, and therefore it is proper to cast all our cares upon Him and rest in His assured providence.

Chapter Two is highlighted with the symbol called **"Akoko Nan Tia Ba Na Onkum Ba"**. It means "God chastises His children to discipline and win them to Himself, not to kill them". It drives the key lesson, that God allows certain hardships and pain in the lives of His children, yet it is His ultimate will to save them and not to destroy them.

Chapter Three has the symbol **"Nyansapo"** which connotes patience, intelligence and wisdom. It is believed that with wisdom, a person can easily know the best means to use in attaining a goal. It has long been the belief of our cultural societies that because God protects and preserves us, all assailants who infiltrate our camp would eventually be overcome through our reliance on knowledge and experience acquired from Him.

Chapter Four has the icon **"Biribi Wo Soro"**, which means "there is a fervent hope that He who is above the skies will send help in time". This must remind us that culturally the right response to challenges in life is not to despair and discard but to remain hopeful and seek help from God. This emblem of hope and inspiration assures us that God watches and listens to us when we pray, and would eventually grant our prayers and aspirations.

The icon for Chapter Five is the symbol **"Adwo"**, which means solitude. Akans believe that having a sense of calm and tranquility within one's self helps to decrease the impact of any turmoil on the outside. Capability to maintain silence in the midst of hardships yields golden results, because quietude overcomes all strife.

Chapter Six has the icon called "**Nyame Nwu Na M'awu**" which is translated as "God Never Dies, Therefore I Will Not Die". This symbolizes faith in God, and the reality that certain challenges/adversities naturally come when we cannot avoid them. But we can salvage what remains and make the most of it. It is therefore proper not to despair, but to reach out with hope and courage for better possibilities.

Chapter Seven's symbolic icon is "**Mmere Dane**". It symbolizes the fleeting nature of time, seasons and all good things in life. It reminds and encourages us that no condition is permanent, hence one ought to exercise humble optimism and eschew anxiety, fear and despair.

The icon for Chapter Eight is "**Nsoromma**". It is the symbol for the star, and it is used to express faith and belief in divine patronage. It is believed that we are children of the Heavens, and we rely on God for every imaginable thing while here on earth.

Chapter Nine has the icon called "**Nyame Adom**", which means in essence that God is gracious. Many events and developments in life point us to the fact that providence abounds. For this reason it is better to count on the promises of God for a good future, than to focus on the mounting challenges of today and be overwhelmed. The belief remains that God has enough resources to share to all who call on Him.

Chapter Ten is highlighted with the symbol called "**Bese Saka**", which means "togetherness breeds unity and affluence. The import of this symbol is that it is prudent to recognize human pain and suffering, and respond with sympathy and support to those who bear the brunt.

Chapter Eleven's icon is "**Osiadan Nyame**". It translates as "God the Builder", and essentially means that God builds all things in His strength and power. He only uses humans as His work tools and material resources. Our recognition of this must humble us and keep us from limiting His abilities or interfering in His purposes. Ours is to trust and cooperate with Him as laborers and tools at His work site.

The icon for Chapter Twelve is "**Eban**". It symbolizes love and security. It is an emblem used to mark out a well secured fortress and homestead where all residents feel protected and free from oppressive forces, discrimination and isolation. This emblem encourages us to believe that God has our backs and He will faithfully keep us safe in Himself.

Ultimately, what is pertinent is that there is a voice with higher authority and greater depth than everything in one's life on earth. This voice is the Holy Spirit who dwells in all who believe in the Lord Jesus Christ. He has the answers to all the puzzles of life, and He has promised to lead us into all truth. Ours is to listen to Him, follow His leading and live in total obedience to His instruction. We cannot go wrong with Him.

REFERENCES

1. **Holy Bible.** New King James Version.

2. William Stillman: **The Autism Answerbook** (Sourcebooks Inc. Illinois; 2007).

3. Linda Dillow: **The Blessing Book** (NavPress, Colorado Springs; 2003)

4. Joni Eareckson Tada: **Glorious Intruder** (Scripture Press, Raans Road Bucks, 1989).

5. Morris Inch: **A Case For Christianity** (1997).

6. Corrie ten Boom: **Marching Orders For The End Battle.** (Christian Literature Crusade, London, 1969).

7. Corrie ten Boom: **Clippings From My Notebook.** (Thomas Nelson Inc. Nashville Tennessee. 1982).

8. Nick Vujicic: **Life Without Limits.** (Doubleday Religion, Random House Inc; New York. 2010).

9. Caren Mayer Cunningham: **Defying Autism.** (Creation House, Florida. 2008)

10. Jan Karon: **Patches Of Godlight.** (Viking Penguin Putnam Inc. Harmondsworth, Middlesex, England, 2001).

11. Matthew Henry: **Commentary On The Whole Bible.** (Marshall, Morgan & Scott Ltd. Zondervan Publishing House, Grand Rapids, Michigan, USA, 1960).

"If you struggle with believing the realism that the Holy Spirit is truly interested in the everyday issues of our lives, and therefore intervenes to direct and provide the wisdom, courage and strength we need to keep going, then this book is for you. You will discover in it real life examples of the Holy Spirit's comforting presence in your life experiences."

By **Nahum Awotwe Ackon**, Businessman, Tema-Ghana.

"Families of autistic children live a life of complexity, faced with stigmatization, scorn, material and emotional costs. Reading this book will make you sensitive to the challenges of living with autism, and provide you a perspective of what support, encouragement and healing you could bring to them. This book is very informative, educating readers on autism and its manifestations in children. It portrays the times and moments in the lives of autistic persons, their parents/family and care-givers. The author shares about the mix of pain, frustration, guilt and sometimes shame in managing autism, and also reveals knowledge and faith in the presence of the Holy Spirit to love, support, instruct and guide His own through it all. It is highly recommended reading for parents, teachers, coaches, nurses, care-givers and all who wish to be helpful neighbours and keepers of our collective humanity".

By **Fred & Evelyn Dimado**, Missionaries, Pioneers International, Thailand.